PAUL KALANITHI

Paul Kalanithi was a neurosurgeon and writer. He held degrees in English literature, human biology, and history and philosophy of science and medicine from Stanford and Cambridge universities before graduating from Yale School of Medicine. He also received the American Academy of Neurological Surgery's highest award for research. His reflections on doctoring and illness have been published in the *New York Times*, the *Washington Post* and the *Paris Review Daily*. Kalanithi died in March 2015, aged 37. He is survived by his wife, Lucy, and their daughter, Elizabeth Acadia.

PAUL KALANITHI

When Breath Becomes Air

FOREWORD BY
Abraham Verghese

VINTAGE

15

Vintage
20 Vauxhall Bridge Road,
London SW1V 2SA

Vintage is part of the Penguin Random House
group of companies whose addresses can be found at
global.penguinrandomhouse.com.

 Penguin
Random House
UK

First published in the UK by The Bodley Head in 2016
First published by Vintage in 2017
This edition published by Vintage in 2018

penguin.co.uk/vintage

A CIP catalogue record for this book
is available from the British Library

ISBN 9781784701994 (B format)
9781529110944 (A format)

Printed and bound in Great Britain by Clays Ltd, Elcograf S.p.A.

Penguin Random House is committed to a sustainable future
for our business, our readers and our planet. This book is made
from Forest Stewardship Council® certified paper.

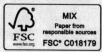

You that seek what life is in death,

Now find it air that once was breath.

New names unknown, old names gone:

Till time end bodies, but souls none.

    Reader! then make time, while you be,

    But steps to your eternity.

—Baron Brooke Fulke Greville, "Caelica 83"

FOREWORD

Abraham Verghese

IT OCCURS TO ME, as I write this, that the foreword to this book might be better thought of as an afterword. Because when it comes to Paul Kalanithi, all sense of time is turned on its head. To begin with—or, maybe, to end with—I got to know Paul only after his death. (Bear with me.) I came to know him most intimately when he'd ceased to be.

I met him one memorable afternoon at Stanford in early February 2014. He'd just published an op-ed titled "How Long Have I Got Left?" in *The New York Times*, an essay that would elicit an overwhelming response, an outpouring from readers. In the ensuing days, it spread exponentially. (I'm an infectious diseases specialist, so please forgive me for not using the word *viral* as a metaphor.) In the aftermath of that, he'd asked to come see me, to chat, to get advice about literary agents, editors, the publishing process—he had a desire to write a book, *this* book, the one you are now holding in your hands. I recall the sun filtering through the magnolia tree outside my office and lighting this scene: Paul seated before me, his beautiful hands exceedingly still, his prophet's beard full, those dark eyes taking the measure of me. In my memory, the picture has a Vermeer-like quality, a camera obscura sharpness. I remember thinking, *You must remember this*, because what was falling on my retina was precious. And because, in the context of Paul's diagnosis, I became aware of not just his mortality but my own.

We talked about a lot of things that afternoon. He was a neurosurgical chief resident. We had probably crossed paths at some point, but we hadn't shared a patient that we could recall. He told me he had been an English and biology major as an undergraduate at Stanford, and then stayed on for a master's in English literature. We talked about his lifelong love of writing and reading. I was struck by how easily he could have been an English professor—and, indeed, he had seemed to be headed down that path at one point in his life. But then, just like his namesake on the road to Damascus, he felt the calling. He became a physician instead, but one who always dreamed of coming back to literature in some form. A book, perhaps. One day. He thought he had time, and why not? And yet now time was the very thing he had so little of.

I remember his wry, gentle smile, a hint of mischief there, even though his face was gaunt and haggard. He'd been through the wringer with this cancer but a new biological therapy had produced a good response, allowing him to look ahead a bit. He said during medical school he'd assumed that he would become a psychiatrist, only to fall in love with neurosurgery. It was much more than a falling in love with the intricacies of the brain, much more than the satisfaction of training his hands to accomplish amazing feats—it was a love and empathy for those who suffered, for what they endured and what he might bring to bear. I don't think he told me this as much as I had heard about this quality of his from students of mine who were his acolytes: his fierce belief in the moral dimension of his job. And then we talked about his dying.

After that meeting, we kept in touch by email, but never saw each other again. It was not just that I disappeared into my own world of deadlines and responsibilities but also my strong sense that the burden was on me to be respectful of his time. It was up to Paul if he wanted to see me. I felt that the last thing he needed was the obligation to service a new friendship. I thought about him a lot, though, and about his wife. I wanted to ask him if he was writing. Was he finding the time? For years, as a busy physician, I'd struggled to find the time to write. I wanted to tell him that a famous writer, commiserating about this eternal problem, once said to me, "If I were a neurosurgeon and I announced that I had to leave my guests to go in for an emergency craniotomy, no one would say a word. But if I said I needed to leave the guests in the living room to go upstairs to *write . . .*" I wondered if Paul would have found this funny. After all, *he* could actually say he was going to do a craniotomy! It was plausible! And then he could go write instead.

While Paul was writing this book, he published a short, remarkable essay in *Stanford Medicine,* in an issue that was devoted to the idea of time. I had an essay in the same issue, my piece juxtaposed to his, though I learned of his contribution only when the magazine was in my hands. In reading his words, I had a second, deeper glimpse of something of which there had been a hint in the *New York Times* essay: Paul's writing was simply stunning. He could have been writing about anything, and it would have been just as powerful. But he *wasn't* writing about anything—he was writing about time and what it meant to him now, in the context of his illness. Which made it all so incredibly poignant.

But here's the thing I must come back to: *the prose was unforgettable*. Out of his pen he was spinning gold.

I reread Paul's piece again and again, trying to understand what he had brought about. First, it was musical. It had echoes of Galway Kinnell, almost a prose poem. ("If one day it happens / you find yourself with someone you love / in a café at one end /of the Pont Mirabeau, at the zinc bar / where wine stands in upward opening glasses . . ." to quote a Kinnell line, from a poem I once heard him recite in a bookstore in Iowa City, never looking down at the paper.) But it also had a taste of something else, something from an antique land, from a time

tion had modern spellings.) The trick, I discovered, was to read it aloud, which made the cadence inescapable: "We carry with us the wonders, we seek without us: There is all Africa, and her prodigies in us; we are that bold and adventurous piece of nature, which he that studies, wisely learns in a compendium, what others labour at in a divided piece and endless volume." When you come to the last paragraph of Paul's book, read it aloud and you will hear that same long line, the cadence you think you can tap your feet to . . . but as with Browne, you will be just off. Paul, it occurred to me, was Browne redux. (Or given that forward time is our illusion, perhaps it's that Browne was Kalanithi redux. Yes, it's head-spinning stuff.)

And then Paul died. I attended his memorial in the Stanford church, a gorgeous space where I often go when it is empty to sit and admire the light, the silence, and where I always find renewal. It was packed for the service. I sat off to one side, listening to a series of moving and sometimes raucous stories from his closest friends, his pastor, and his brother. Yes, Paul was gone, but strangely, I felt I was coming to know him, beyond that visit in my office, beyond the few essays he'd written. He was taking form in those tales being told in the Stanford Memorial Church, its soaring cathedral dome a fitting space in which to remember this man whose body was now in the earth but who nevertheless was so palpably *alive*. He took form in the shape of his lovely wife and baby daughter, his grieving parents and siblings, in the faces of the legions of friends, colleagues, and former patients who filled that space; he was there at the reception later, outdoors in a setting where so many came together. I saw faces looking calm, smiling, as if they had witnessed something profoundly beautiful in the church. Perhaps my face was like that, too: we had found meaning in the ritual of a service, in the ritual of eulogizing, in the shared tears. There was further meaning residing in this reception where we slaked our thirst, fed our bodies, and talked with complete strangers to whom we were intimately connected through Paul.

But it was only when I received the pages that you now hold in your hands, two months after Paul died, that I felt I had finally come to know him, to know him better than if I had been blessed to call him a friend. After reading the book you are about to read, I confess I felt inadequate: there was an honesty, a truth in the writing that took my breath away.

Be ready. Be seated. See what courage sounds like. See how brave it is to reveal yourself in this way. But above all, see what it is to still live, to profoundly influence the lives of others after you are gone, by your words. In a world of asynchronous communication, where we are so often buried in our screens, our gaze rooted to the rectangular objects buzzing in our hands, our attention consumed by ephemera, stop and experience this dialogue with my young departed colleague, now ageless and extant in memory. Listen to Paul. In the silences between his words, listen to what you have to say back. Therein lies his message. I got it. I hope you experience it, too. It is a gift. Let me not stand between you and Paul.

CONTENTS

WHEN BREATH
BECOMES AIR

PROLOGUE

Webster was much possessed by death
And saw the skull beneath the skin;
And breastless creatures under ground
Leaned backward with a lipless grin.

—T. S. Eliot, "Whispers of Immortality"

I FLIPPED THROUGH THE CT scan images, the diagnosis obvious: the lungs were matted with innumerable tumors, the spine deformed, a full lobe of the liver obliterated. Cancer, widely disseminated. I was a neurosurgical resident entering my final year of training. Over the last six years, I'd examined scores of such scans, on the off chance that some procedure might benefit the patient. But this scan was different: it was my own.

I wasn't in the radiology suite, wearing my scrubs and white coat. I was dressed in a patient's gown, tethered to an IV pole, using the computer the nurse had left in my hospital room, with my wife, Lucy, an internist, at my side. I went through each sequence again: the lung window, the bone window, the liver window, scrolling from top to bottom, then left to right, then front to back, just as I had been trained to do, as if I might find something that would change the diagnosis.

We lay together on the hospital bed.

Lucy, quietly, as if reading from a script: "Do you think there's any possibility that it's something else?"

"No," I said.

We held each other tightly, like young lovers. In the past year we'd both suspected, but refused to believe, or even discuss, that a cancer was growing inside me.

About six months before, I had started losing weight and having ferocious back pain. When I dressed in the morning, my belt cinched one, then two notches tighter. I went to see my primary care doctor, an old classmate from Stanford. Her sister had died suddenly as a neurosurgery intern, after contracting a virulent infection, and so she'd taken a maternal watch on my health. When I arrived, however, I found a different doctor in her office—my classmate was on maternity leave.

Dressed in a thin blue gown on a cold examining table, I described the symptoms to her. "Of course," I meek in a patient's gown? The truth was, I knew more about back pain than she did—half of my training as a neurosurgeon had involved disorders of the spine. But maybe a spondy *was* more likely. It did affect a significant percent of young adults—and cancer in the spine in your thirties? The odds of that couldn't be more than one in ten thousand. Even if it were one hundred times more common than that, it'd still be less common than a spondy. Maybe I was just freaking myself out.

The X-rays looked fine. We chalked the symptoms up to hard work and an aging body, scheduled a follow-up appointment, and I went back to finish my last case of the day. The weight loss slowed, and the back pain became tolerable. A healthy dose of ibuprofen got me through the day, and after all, there weren't that many of these grueling, fourteen-hour days left. My journey from medical student to professor of neurosurgery was almost complete: after ten years of relentless training, I was determined to persevere for the next fifteen months, until residency ended. I had earned the respect of my seniors, won prestigious national awards, and was fielding job offers from several major universities. My program director at Stanford had recently sat me down and said,

"Paul, I think you'll be the number one candidate for any job you apply for. Just as an FYI: we'll be starting a faculty search for someone like you here. No promises, of course, but it's something you should consider."

At age thirty-six, I had reached the mountaintop; I could see the Promised Land, from Gilead to Jericho to the Mediterranean Sea. I could see a nice catamaran on that sea that Lucy, our hypothetical children, and I would take out on weekends. I could see the tension in my back unwinding as my work schedule eased and life became more manageable. I could see myself finally becoming the husband I'd promised to be.

Then, a few weeks later, I began having bouts of severe chest pain. Had I bumped into something at work? Cracked a rib somehow? Some nights, I'd wake up on soaked sheets, dripping sweat. My weight began dropping again, more rapidly now, from 175 to 145 pounds. I developed a persistent cough. Little doubt remained. One Saturday afternoon, Lucy and I were lying in the sun in Dolores Park in San Francisco, waiting to meet her sister. She glimpsed my phone screen, which displayed medical database search results: "frequency of cancers in thirty- to forty-year-olds."

time to consider the state of our marriage. She spoke in even tones, which only heightened the vertigo I felt.

"What?" I said. "No."

"I love you so much, which is why this is so confusing," she said. "But I'm worried we want different things from our relationship. I feel like we're connected halfway. I don't want to learn about your worries by accident. When I talk to you about feeling isolated, you don't seem to think it's a problem. I need to do something different."

"Things are going to be okay," I said. "It's just residency."

Were things really so bad? Neurosurgical training, among the most rigorous and demanding of all medical specialties, had surely put a strain on our marriage. There were so many nights when I came home late from work, after Lucy had gone to bed, and collapsed on the living room floor, exhausted, and so many mornings when I left for work in the early dark, before she'd awoken. But our careers were peaking now—most universities wanted both of us: me in neurosurgery, Lucy in internal medicine. We'd survived the most difficult part of our journey. Hadn't we discussed this a dozen times?

Didn't she realize this was the worst possible time for her to blow things up? Didn't she see that I had only one year left in residency, that I loved her, that we were so close to the life together we'd always wanted?

"If it were just residency, I could make it," she said. "We've made it this far. But the problem is, what if it's *not* just residency? Do you really think things will be better when you're an academic neurosurgery attending?"

I offered to skip the trip, to be more open, to see the couples therapist Lucy had suggested a few months ago, but she insisted that she needed time—alone. At that point, the fuzziness of the confusion dissipated, leaving only a hard edge. Fine, I said. If she decided to leave, then I would assume the relationship was over. If it turned out that I had cancer, I wouldn't tell her—she'd be free to live whatever life she chose.

Before leaving for New York, I snuck in a few medical appointments to rule out some common cancers in the young. (Testicular? No. Melanoma? No. Leukemia? No.) The neurosurgical service was busy, as always. Thursday night slipped into Friday morning as I was caught in the operating room for thirty-six hours straight, in a series of deeply complex cases: giant aneurysms, intracerebral arterial bypasses, arteriovenous malformations. I breathed a silent thanks when the attending came in, allowing me a few minutes to ease my back against a wall. The only time to get a chest X-ray was as I was leaving the hospital, on the way home before heading to the airport. I figured either I had cancer, in which case this might be the last time I would see my friends, or I didn't, in which case there was no reason to cancel the trip.

I rushed home to grab my bags. Lucy drove me to the airport and told me she had scheduled us into couples therapy.

From the gate, I sent her a text message: "I wish you were here."

A few minutes later, the response came back: "I love you. I will be here when you get back."

My back stiffened terribly during the flight, and by the time I made it to Grand Central to catch a train to my friends' place upstate, my body was rippling with pain. Over the past few months, I'd had back spasms of varying ferocity, from simple ignorable pain, to pain that made me forsake speech to grind my teeth, to pain so severe I curled up on the floor, screaming. This pain was toward the more severe end of the spectrum. I lay down on a hard bench in the waiting area, feeling my back muscles contort, breathing to control the pain—the ibuprofen wasn't touching this—and naming each muscle as it spasmed to stave off tears: erector spinae, rhomboid, latissimus, piriformis . . .

A security guard approached. "Sir, you can't lie down here."

"I'm sorry," I said, gasping out the words. "Bad . . . back . . . spasms."

"You still can't lie down here."

I'm sorry, but I'm dying from cancer.

The words lingered on my tongue—but what if I wasn't? Maybe this was just what people with back pain live with. I knew a lot about back pain—its anatomy, its physiology, the different words patients used to describe different kinds of pain—but I didn't know what it *felt* like. Maybe that's all this was. Maybe. Or maybe I didn't want the jinx. Maybe I just didn't want to say the word *cancer* out loud.

I pulled myself up and hobbled to the platform.

It was late afternoon when I reached the house in Cold Spring, fifty miles north of Manhattan on the Hudson River, and was greeted by a dozen of my closest friends from years past, their cheers of welcome mixed with the cacophony of young, happy children. Hugs ensued, and an ice-cold dark and stormy made its way to my hand.

"No Lucy?"

"Sudden work thing," I said. "Very last-minute."

"Oh, what a bummer!"

"Say, do you mind if I put my bags down and rest a bit?"

I had hoped a few days out of the OR, with adequate sleep, rest, and relaxation—in short, a taste of a normal life—would bring my symptoms back into the normal spectrum for back pain and fatigue. But after a day or two, it was clear there would be no reprieve.

I slept through breakfasts and shambled to the lunch table to stare at ample plates of cassoulet and crab legs that I couldn't bring myself to eat. By dinner, I was exhausted, ready for bed again. Sometimes I read to the kids, but mostly they played on and around me, leaping and yelling. ("Kids, I think Uncle Paul needs a rest. Why don't you play over there?") I remembered a day off as a summer camp counselor, fifteen years prior, sitting on the shore of a lake in Northern California, with a bunch of joyous kids using me as an obstacle in a convoluted game of Capture the Flag, while I read a book called *Death and Philosophy*. I used to laugh at the incongruities of that moment: a twenty-year-old amid the splendor of trees, lake, mountains, the chirping of birds mixed with the squeal of happy four-year-olds, his nose buried in a small black book about death. Only now, in this moment, I felt the parallels: instead of Lake Tahoe, it was the Hudson River; the children were not strangers', but my friends'; instead of a book on death separating me from the life around me, it was my own body, dying.

On the third night, I spoke to Mike, our host, to tell him I was going to cut the trip short and head home the next day.

"You don't look so great," he said. "Everything okay?"

"Why don't we grab some scotch and have a seat?" I said.

In front of his fireplace, I said, "Mike, I think I have cancer. And not the good kind, either."

It was the first time I'd said it out loud.

"Okay," he said. "I take it this is not some elaborate practical joke?"

"No."

He paused. "I don't know exactly what to ask."

"Well, I suppose, first, I should say that I don't know for a *fact* that I have cancer. I'm just pretty sure of it—a lot of the symptoms point that way. I'm going to go home tomorrow and sort it out. Hopefully, I'm wrong."

Mike offered to take my luggage and send it home by mail, so I wouldn't have to carry it with me. He drove me to the airport early the next morning, and six hours later I landed in San Francisco. My phone rang as I stepped off the plane. It was my primary care doctor, calling with the chest X-ray result: my lungs, instead of being clear, looked blurry, as if the camera aperture had been left open too long. The doctor said she wasn't sure what that meant.

She likely knew what it meant.

I knew.

Lucy picked me up from the airport, but I waited until we were home to tell her. We sat on the couch, and when I told her, she knew. She leaned her head on my shoulder, and the distance between us vanished.

"I need you," I whispered.

"I will never leave you," she said.

We called a close friend, one of the attending neuro-surgeons at the hospital, and asked him to admit me.

I received the plastic arm bracelet all patients wear, put on the familiar light blue hospital gown, walked past the nurses I knew by name, and was checked in to a room—the same room where I had seen hundreds of patients over the years. In this room, I had sat with patients and explained terminal diagnoses and complex operations; in this room, I had congratulated patients on being cured of a disease and seen their happiness at being returned to their lives; in this room, I had pronounced patients dead. I had sat in the chairs, washed my hands in the sink, scrawled instructions on the marker board, changed the calendar. I had even, in moments of utter exhaustion, longed to lie down in this bed and sleep. Now I lay there, wide awake.

A young nurse, one I hadn't met, poked her head in.

"The doctor will be in soon."

And with that, the future I had imagined, the one just about to be realized, the culmination of decades of striving, evaporated.

PART I

In Perfect Health I Begin

> The hand of the LORD was upon me, and carried me out in the
> spirit of the LORD, and set me down in the midst of the valley
> which was full of bones,
>
> And caused me to pass by them round about: and, behold, there
> were very many in the open valley; and, lo, they were very
> dry.
>
> And he said unto me, Son of man, can these bones live?
>
> —Ezekiel 37:1–3, King James translation

I KNEW WITH CERTAINTY that I would never be a doctor. I stretched out in the sun, relaxing on a desert plateau just above our house. My uncle, a doctor, like so many of my relatives, had asked me earlier that day what I planned on doing for a career, now that I was heading off to college, and the question barely registered. If you had forced me to answer, I suppose I would have said a writer, but frankly, thoughts of any career at this point seemed absurd. I was leaving this small Arizona town in a few weeks, and I felt less like someone preparing to climb a career ladder than a buzzing electron about to achieve escape velocity, flinging out into a strange and sparkling universe.

I lay there in the dirt, awash in sunlight and memory, feeling the shrinking size of this town of fifteen thousand, six hundred miles from my new college dormitory at Stanford and all its promise.

I knew medicine only by its absence—specifically, the absence of a father growing up, one who went to work before dawn and returned in the dark to a plate of reheated dinner. When I was ten, my father had moved us—three boys, ages fourteen, ten, and eight—from Bronxville, New York, a compact, affluent suburb just north of Manhattan, to Kingman, Arizona, in a desert valley ringed by two mountain ranges, known primarily to the outside world as a place to get gas en route to somewhere else. He was drawn by the sun, by the cost of living—how else would he pay for his sons to attend the colleges he aspired to?—and by the opportunity to establish a regional cardiology practice of his own. His unyielding dedication to his patients soon made him a respected member of the community. When we did see him, late at night or on weekends, he was an amalgam of sweet affections and austere diktats, hugs and kisses mixed with stony pronouncements: "It's very easy to be number one: find the guy who is number one, and score one point higher than he does." He had reached some compromise in his mind that fatherhood could be distilled; short, concentrated (but sincere) bursts of high intensity could equal ... whatever it was that other fathers did. All I knew was, if that was the price of medicine, it was simply too high.

From my desert plateau, I could see our house, just beyond the city limits, at the base of the Cerbat Mountains, amid red-rock desert speckled with mesquite, tumbleweeds, and paddle-shaped cacti. Out here, dust devils swirled up from nothing, blurring your vision, then disappeared. Spaces stretched on, then fell away into the distance. Our two dogs, Max and Nip, never grew tired of the freedom. Every day, they'd venture forth and bring home some new desert treasure: the leg of a deer, unfinished bits of jackrabbit to eat later, the sun-bleached skull of a horse, the jawbone of a coyote.

My friends and I loved the freedom, too, and we spent our afternoons exploring, walking, scavenging for bones and rare desert creeks. Having spent my previous years in a lightly forested suburb in the Northeast, with a tree-lined main street and a candy store, I found the wild, windy desert alien and alluring. On my first trek alone, as a ten-year-old, I discovered an old irrigation grate. I pried it open with my fingers, lifted it up, and there, a few inches from my face, were three white silken webs, and in each, marching along on spindled legs, was a glistening black bulbous body, bearing in its shine the dreaded blood-red hourglass. Near to each spider a pale, pulsating sac breathed with the imminent birth of countless more black widows. Horror let the grate crash shut. I stumbled back. The horror came in a mix of "country facts" (*Nothing is more deadly than the bite of the black widow spider*) and the inhuman posture and the black shine and the red hourglass. I had nightmares for years.

The desert offered a pantheon of terrors: tarantulas, wolf spiders, fiddlebacks, bark scorpions, whip scorpions, centipedes, diamondbacks, sidewinders, Mojave greens. Eventually we grew familiar, even comfortable, with these creatures. For fun, when my friends and I discovered a wolf spider's nest, we'd drop an ant onto its outer limits and watch as its entangled escape attempts sent quivers down the silk strands, into the spider's dark central hole, anticipating that fatal moment when the spider would burst from its hollows and seize the doomed ant in its mandibles. "Country facts" became my term for the rural cousin of the urban legend. As I first learned them, country facts granted fairy powers to desert creatures, making, say, the Gila monster no less an actual monster than the Gorgon. Only after living out in the desert for a while did we realize that some country facts, like the existence of the jackalope, had been deliberately created to confuse city folk and amuse the locals. I once spent an hour convincing a group of exchange students from Berlin that, yes, there *was* a particular species of coyote that lived inside cacti and could leap ten yards to attack its prey (like, well, unsuspecting Germans). Yet no one precisely knew where the truth lay amid the whirling sand; for every country fact that seemed preposterous, there was one that felt solid and true. *Always check your shoes for scorpions*, for example, seemed plain good sense.

When I was sixteen, I was supposed to drive my younger brother, Jeevan, to school. One morning, as usual, I was running late, and as Jeevan was standing impatiently in the foyer, yelling that he didn't want to get detention again because of my tardiness, so could I please hurry the hell up, I raced down the stairs, threw open the front door . . . and nearly stepped on a snoozing six-foot rattlesnake. It was another country fact that if you killed a rattlesnake on your doorstep, its mate and offspring would come and make a permanent nest there, like Grendel's mother seeking her revenge. So Jeevan and I drew straws: the lucky one grabbed a shovel, the unlucky one a pair of thick gardening gloves and a pillowcase, and through a seriocomic dance, we managed to get the snake into the pillowcase. Then, like an Olympic hammer thrower, I hurled the whole out into the desert, with plans to retrieve the pillowcase later that afternoon, so as not to get in trouble with our mother.

Of our many childhood mysteries, chief among them was not why our father decided to bring his family to the desert town of Kingman, Arizona, which we grew to cherish, but how he ever convinced my mother to join him there. They had eloped, in love, across the world, from southern India to New York City (he a Christian, she a Hindu, their marriage was condemned on both sides, and led to years of familial rifts—my mother's mother never acknowledged my name, Paul, instead insisting I be called by my middle name, Sudhir) to Arizona, where my mother was forced to confront an intractable mortal fear of snakes. Even the smallest, cutest, most harmless red racer would send her screaming into the house, where she'd lock the doors and arm herself with the nearest large, sharp implement—rake, cleaver, ax.

The snakes were a constant source of anxiety, but it was her children's future that my mother feared for most of all. Before we moved, my older brother, Suman, had nearly completed high school in Westchester County, where elite colleges were the expectation. He was accepted to Stanford shortly after arriving in Kingman and left the house soon thereafter. But Kingman, we learned, was not Westchester. As my mother surveyed the Mohave County public school system, she became distraught. The U.S. census had recently identified Kingman as the least educated district in America. The high school dropout rate was somewhere north of 30 percent. Few students went on to college, and certainly none to Harvard, my father's standard of excellence. Looking for advice, my mother called her friends and relatives from wealthy East Coast suburbs and found some sympathetic, others gleeful that their children no longer had to compete with the suddenly education-starved Kalanithis.

At night, she broke into tears, sobbing alone in her bed. My mother, afraid the impoverished school system would hobble her children, acquired, from somewhere, a "college prep reading list." Trained in India to be a physiologist, married at twenty-three, and preoccupied with raising three kids in a country that was not her own, she had not read many of the books on the list herself. But she would make sure her kids were not deprived. She made me read *1984* when I was ten years old; I was scandalized by the sex, but it also instilled in me a deep love of, and care for, language.

Endless books and authors followed, as we worked our way methodically down the list: *The Count of Monte Cristo*, Edgar Allan Poe, *Robinson Crusoe*, *Ivanhoe*, Gogol, *The Last of the Mohicans*, Dickens, Twain, Austen, *Billy Budd* . . . By the time I was twelve, I was picking them out myself, and my brother Suman was sending me the books he had read in college: *The Prince*, *Don Quixote*, *Candide*, *Le Morte D'Arthur*, *Beowulf*, Thoreau, Sartre,

Camus. Some left more of a mark than others. *Brave New World* founded my nascent moral philosophy and became the subject of my college admissions essay, in which I argued that happiness was not the point of life. *Hamlet* bore me a thousand times through the usual adolescent crises. "To His Coy Mistress" and other romantic poems led me and my friends on various joyful misadventures throughout high school—we often sneaked out at night to, for example, sing "American Pie" beneath the window of the captain of the cheerleading team. (Her father was a local minister and so, we reasoned, less likely to shoot.) After I was caught returning at dawn from one such late-night escapade, my worried mother thoroughly interrogated me regarding every drug teenagers take, never suspecting that the most intoxicating thing I'd experienced, by far, was the volume of romantic poetry she'd handed me the previous week. Books became my closest confidants, finely ground lenses providing new views of the world.

In her quest to see that her children were educated, my mom drove us more than a hundred miles north, to the nearest big city, Las Vegas, so we could take our PSATs, SATs, and ACTs. She joined the school board, rallied teachers, and demanded that AP classes be added to the curriculum. She was a phenom: she took it upon herself to transform the Kingman school system, and she did. Suddenly there was a feeling in our high school that the two mountain ranges that bounded the town no longer defined the horizon: it was what lay beyond them.

Senior year, my close friend Leo, our salutatorian and the poorest kid I knew, was advised by the school guidance counselor, "You're smart—you should join the army."

He told me about it afterward. "Fuck that," he said. "If *you're* going to Harvard, or Yale, or Stanford, then I am, too."

I don't know if I was happier when I got into Stanford or when Leo got into Yale.

Summer passed, and since Stanford began classes a month later than every other school, all of my friends scattered, leaving me behind. Most afternoons, I'd trek into the desert alone and nap and think until my girlfriend, Abigail, got off her shift at Kingman's lone coffee shop. The desert offered a shortcut, through the mountains and down into town, and hiking was more fun than driving. Abigail was in her early twenties, a student at

Scripps College who, wanting to avoid loans, was taking a semester off to stockpile tuition money. I was taken with her worldliness, the sense that she knew secrets one only learned at college—she had studied psychology!—and we'd often meet as she got off work. She was a harbinger of the *sub rosa*, the new world awaiting me in just a few weeks. One afternoon, I woke from my nap, looked up, and saw vultures circling, mistaking me for carrion. I checked my watch; it was almost three. I was going to be late. I dusted off my jeans and jogged the rest of the way through the desert, until sand gave way to pavement, the first buildings appeared, and I rounded the corner to find Abigail, broom in hand, sweeping the coffee shop deck.

"I already cleaned the espresso machine," she said, "so no iced latte for you today."

The floors swept, we went inside. Abigail walked to the cash register and picked up a paperback she'd stashed there. "Here," she said, tossing it at me. "You should read this. You're always reading such high-culture crap—why don't you try something lowbrow for once?"

It was a five-hundred-page novel called *Satan: His Psychotherapy and Cure by the Unfortunate Dr. Kassler,*

J.S.P.S., by Jeremy Leven. I took it home and read it in a day. It wasn't high culture. It should have been funny, but it wasn't. However, it did make the throwaway assumption that the mind was simply the operation of the brain, an idea that struck me with force; it startled my naïve understanding of the world. Of course, it must be true—what were our brains doing, otherwise? Though we had free will, we were also biological organisms—the brain was an organ, subject to all the laws of physics, too! Literature provided a rich account of human meaning; the brain, then, was the machinery that somehow enabled it. It seemed like magic. That night, in my room, I opened up my red Stanford course catalog, which I had read through dozens of times, and grabbed a highlighter. In addition to all the literature classes I had marked, I began looking in biology and neuroscience as well.

A few years later, I hadn't thought much more about a career but had nearly completed degrees in English literature and human biology. I was driven less by achievement than by trying to understand, in earnest: What makes human life meaningful? I still felt literature provided the best account of the life of the mind, while neuroscience laid down the most elegant rules of the brain. Meaning, while a slippery concept, seemed inextricable from human relationships and moral values. T. S. Eliot's *The Waste Land* resonated profoundly, relating meaninglessness and isolation, and the desperate quest for human connection. I found Eliot's metaphors leaking into my own language. Other authors resonated as well. Nabokov, for his awareness of how our suffering can make us callous to the obvious suffering of another. Conrad, for his hypertuned sense of how miscommunication between people can so profoundly impact their lives. Literature not only illuminated another's experience, it provided, I believed, the richest material for moral reflection. My brief forays into the formal ethics of analytic philosophy felt dry as a bone, missing the messiness and weight of real human life.

Throughout college, my monastic, scholarly study of human meaning would conflict with my urge to forge and strengthen the human relationships that formed that meaning. If the unexamined life was not worth living, was the unlived life worth examining? Heading into my sophomore summer, I applied for two jobs: as an intern at the highly scientific Yerkes Primate Research Center, in Atlanta, and as a prep chef at Sierra Camp, a family vacation spot for Stanford alumni on the pristine shores of Fallen Leaf Lake, abutting the stark beauty of Desolation Wilderness in Eldorado National Forest. The camp's literature promised, simply, the best summer of your life. I was surprised and flattered to be accepted. Yet I had just learned that macaques had a rudimentary form of culture, and I was eager to go to Yerkes and see what could be the natural origin of meaning itself. In other words, I could either study meaning or I could experience it.

After delaying for as long as possible, I finally chose the camp. Afterward, I dropped by my biology adviser's office to inform him of my decision. When I walked in, he was sitting at his desk, head in a journal, as usual. He was a quiet, amiable man with heavy-lidded eyes, but as I told him my plans, he became a different person entirely: his eyes shot open, and his face flushed red, flecks of spit spraying.

"What?" he said. "When you grow up, are you going to be a scientist or a . . . *chef*?"

Eventually the term ended and I was on the windy

mountain road to camp, still slightly worried that I'd made a wrong turn in life. My doubt, however, was short-lived. The camp delivered on its promise, concentrating all the idylls of youth: beauty manifest in lakes, mountains, people; richness in experience, conversation, friendships. Nights during a full moon, the light flooded the wilderness, so it was possible to hike without a headlamp. We would hit the trail at two A.M., summiting the nearest peak, Mount Tallac, just before sunrise, the clear, starry night reflected in the flat, still lakes spread below us. Snuggled together in sleeping bags at the peak, nearly ten thousand feet up, we weathered frigid blasts of wind with coffee someone had been thoughtful enough to bring. And then we would sit and watch as the first hint of sunlight, a light tinge of day blue, would leak out of the eastern horizon, slowly erasing the stars. The day sky would spread wide and high, until the first ray of the sun made an appearance. The morning commuters began to animate the distant South Lake Tahoe roads. But craning your head back, you could see the day's blue darken halfway across the sky, and to the west, the night remained yet unconquered—pitch-black, stars in full glimmer, the full moon still pinned in the sky. To the

amongst the driftwood, my teeth amongst the sand. . . . I don't believe in the wisdom of children, nor in the wisdom of the old. There is a moment, a cusp, when the sum of gathered experience is worn down by the details of living. We are never so wise as when we live in this moment.

Back on campus, I didn't miss the monkeys. Life felt rich and full, and over the next two years I kept at it, seeking a deeper understanding of a life of the mind. I studied literature and philosophy to understand what makes life meaningful, studied neuroscience and worked in an fMRI lab to understand how the brain could give rise to an organism capable of finding meaning in the world, and enriched my relationships with a circle of dear friends through various escapades. We raided the school cafeteria dressed as Mongols; created a full fake fraternity, complete with fake rush-week events, in our co-op house; posed in front of the gates at Buckingham Palace in a gorilla suit; broke into Memorial Church at midnight to lie on our backs and listen to our voices echo in the apse; and so on. (Then I learned that Virginia Woolf once boarded a battleship dressed as Abyssinian royalty, and, duly chastened, stopped boasting about our trivial pranks.)

Senior year, in one of my last neuroscience classes, on neuroscience and ethics, we visited a home for people who had suffered severe brain injuries. We walked into the main reception area and were greeted by a disconsolate wailing. Our guide, a friendly thirty-something woman, introduced herself to the group, but my eyes hunted for the source of the noise. Behind the reception counter was a large-screen television showing a soap opera, on mute. A blue-eyed brunette with well-coiffed hair, her head shaking slightly with emotion, filled the screen as she pleaded with someone off camera; zoom out, and there was her strong-jawed, undoubtedly gravel-voiced lover; they embraced passionately. The wailing rose in pitch. I stepped closer to peer over the counter, and there, on a blue mat in front of the television, in a plain flower-print dress, was a young woman, maybe twenty, her hands balled into fists pressed into her eyes, violently rocking back and forth, wailing and wailing. As she rocked, I caught glimpses of the back of her head, where her hair had worn away, leaving a large, pale patch of skin.

I stepped back to join the group, which was leaving to tour the facility. Talking with the guide, I learned that many of the residents had nearly drowned as young children. Looking around, I noticed there were no other visitors besides us. Was that common? I asked.

At first, the guide explained, a family will visit constantly, daily or even twice a day. Then maybe every other day. Then just weekends. After months or years, the visits taper off, until it's just, say, birthdays and Christmas. Eventually, most families move away, as far as they can get.

"I don't blame them," she said. "It's hard caring for these kids."

A fury churned in me. *Hard?* Of course it was hard, but how could parents abandon these kids? In one room, the patients lay on cots, mostly still, arranged in neat rows like soldiers in a barracks. I walked down a row until I made eye contact with one of them. She was in her late teens, with dark, tangled hair. I paused and tried smiling at her, showing her I cared. I picked up one of her hands; it was limp. But she gurgled and, looking right at me, smiled.

"I think she's smiling," I said to the attendant.

"Could be," she said. "It can be hard to tell sometimes."

But I was sure of it. She was smiling.

When we got back to campus, I was the last one left in the room with the professor. "So, what'd you think?" he asked.

I vented openly about how I couldn't believe that parents had abandoned these poor kids, and how one of them had even smiled at me.

The professor was a mentor, someone who thought deeply about how science and morality intersected. I expected him to agree with me.

"Yeah," he said. "Good. Good for you. But sometimes, you know, I think it's better if they die."

I grabbed my bag and left.

She *had* been smiling, hadn't she?

Only later would I realize that our trip had added a new dimension to my understanding of the fact that brains give rise to our ability to form relationships and make life meaningful. Sometimes, they break.

...

As graduation loomed, I had a nagging sense that there was still far too much unresolved for me, that I wasn't done studying. I applied for a master's in English literature at Stanford and was accepted into the program. I had come to see language as an almost supernatural force, existing between people, bringing our brains, shielded in centimeter-thick skulls, into communion. A word meant something only between people, and life's meaning, its virtue, had something to do with the depth of the relationships we form. It was the relational aspect of humans—i.e., "human relationality"—that undergirded meaning. Yet somehow, this process existed in brains and bodies, subject to their own physiologic imperatives, prone to breaking and failing. There must be a way, I thought, that the language of life as experienced—of passion, of hunger, of love—bore some relationship, however convoluted, to the language of neurons, digestive tracts, and heartbeats.

At Stanford, I had the good fortune to study with Richard Rorty, perhaps the greatest living philosopher of his day, and under his tutelage I began to see all disciplines as creating a vocabulary, a set of tools for understanding human life in a particular way. Great literary works provided their own sets of tools, compelling the reader to use that vocabulary. For my thesis, I studied the work of Walt Whitman, a poet who, a century before, was possessed by the same questions that haunted me, who wanted to find a way to understand and describe what he termed "the Physiological-Spiritual Man."

As I finished my thesis, I could only conclude that Whitman had had no better luck than the rest of us at building a coherent "physiological-spiritual" vocabulary, but at least the ways in which he'd failed were illuminating. I was also increasingly certain that I had little desire to continue in literary studies, whose main preoccupations had begun to strike me as overly political and averse to science. One of my thesis advisers remarked that finding a community for myself in the literary world would be difficult, because most English PhDs reacted to science, as he put it, "like apes to fire, with sheer terror." I wasn't sure where my life was headed. My thesis—"Whitman and the Medicalization of Personality"—was well-received, but it was unorthodox, including as much history of psychiatry and neuroscience as literary criticism. It didn't quite fit in an English department. *I* didn't quite fit in an English department.

Some of my closest friends from college were headed to New York City to pursue a life in the arts—some in comedy, others in journalism and television—and I briefly considered joining them and starting anew. But I couldn't quite let go of the question: Where did biology, morality, literature, and philosophy intersect? Walking home from a football game one afternoon, the autumn breeze blowing, I let my mind wander. Augustine's voice in the garden commanded, "Take up and read," but the voice I heard commanded the opposite: "Set aside the books and practice medicine." Suddenly, it all seemed obvious. Although—or perhaps because—my father, my uncle, and my elder brother were all doctors, medicine had never occurred to me as a serious possibility. But hadn't Whitman himself written that only the physician could truly understand "the Physiological-Spiritual Man"?

The next day, I consulted a premed adviser to figure out the logistics. Getting ready for medical school would take about a year of intense coursework, plus the application time, which added up to another eighteen months. It would mean letting my friends go to New York, to continue deepening those relationships, without me. It would mean setting aside literature. But it would allow me a chance to find answers that are not in books, to find a different sort of sublime, to forge relationships with the suffering, and to keep following the question of what makes human life meaningful, even in the face of death and decay.

I began working through the necessary premedical courses, loading up on chemistry and physics. Reluctant to take a part-time job—it would slow my studies—but unable to afford Palo Alto rent, I found an open window in an empty dormitory and climbed in. After a few weeks of squatting, I was discovered by the caretaker—who happened to be a friend. She provided a key to the room and some useful warnings, like when the high school girls' cheerleading camps would be coming through. Thinking it wise to avoid becoming a registered sex offender, I'd pack a tent, some books and granola, and head up to Tahoe until it was safe to return.

Because the med school application cycle takes eighteen months, I had a free year once my classes were over.

Several professors had suggested I pursue a degree in the history and philosophy of science and medicine before deciding to leave academia for good. So I applied for, and was accepted into, the HPS program at Cambridge. I spent the next year in classrooms in the English countryside, where I found myself increasingly often arguing that direct experience of life-and-death questions was essential to generating substantial moral opinions about them. Words began to feel as weightless as the breath that carried them. Stepping back, I realized that I was merely confirming what I already knew: I wanted that direct experience. It was only in practicing medicine that I could pursue a serious biological philosophy. Moral speculation was puny compared to moral action. I finished my degree and headed back to the States. I was going to Yale for medical school.

You would think that the first time you cut up a dead person, you'd feel a bit funny about it. Strangely, though, everything feels normal. The bright lights, stainless steel tables, and bow-tied professors lend an air of propriety. Even so, that first cut, running from the nape of the neck down to the small of the back, is unforgettable. The scalpel is so sharp it doesn't so much cut the skin as unzip it, revealing the hidden and forbidden sinew beneath, and despite your preparation, you are caught unawares, ashamed and excited. Cadaver dissection is a medical rite of passage and a trespass on the sacrosanct, engendering a legion of feelings: from revulsion, exhilaration, nausea, frustration, and awe to, as time passes, the mere tedium of academic exercise. Everything teeters between pathos and bathos: here you are, violating society's most fundamental taboos, and yet formaldehyde is a powerful appetite stimulant, so you also crave a burrito. Eventually, as you complete your assignments by dissecting the median nerve, sawing the pelvis in half, and slicing open the heart, the bathos supersedes: the sacred violation takes on the character of your average college class, replete with pedants, class clowns, and the rest. Cadaver dissection epitomizes, for many, the transformation of the somber, respectful student into the callous, arrogant doctor.

The enormity of the moral mission of medicine lent my early days of med school a severe gravity. The first day, before we got to the cadavers, was CPR training, my second time doing it. The first time, back in college, had been farcical, unserious, everyone laughing: the terribly acted videos and limbless plastic mannequins couldn't have been more artificial. But now the lurking possibility that we would have to employ these skills someday animated everything. As I repeatedly slammed my palm into the chest of a tiny plastic child, I couldn't help but hear, along with my fellow students' jokes, real ribs cracking.

Cadavers reverse the polarity. The mannequins you pretend are real; the cadavers you pretend are fake. But that first day, you just can't. When I faced my cadaver, slightly blue and bloated, his total deadness and total humanness were undeniable. The knowledge that in four months I would be bisecting this man's head with a hacksaw seemed unconscionable.

Yet there are anatomy professors. And the advice they gave us was to take one good look at our cadaver's face and then leave it covered; it makes the work easier. Just as we prepared, with deep breaths and earnest looks, to unwrap our cadaver's head, a surgeon stopped by to chat, leaning with his elbows on the corpse's face. Pointing out various marks and scars on the naked torso, he reconstructed the patient's history. This scar is from an inguinal hernia operation, this one a carotid endarterectomy; these marks here indicate scratching, possibly jaundice, high bilirubin; he probably died of pancreatic cancer, though no scar for that—killed him too quick. Meanwhile, I could not help but stare at the shifting elbows that, with each medical hypothesis and vocabulary lesson, rolled over this covered head. I thought: *Prosopagnosia is a neurological disorder wherein one loses the ability to see faces.* Pretty soon I would have it, hacksaw in hand.

Because after a few weeks, the drama dissipated. In conversations with non–medical students, telling cadaver stories, I found myself highlighting the grotesque, macabre, and absurd, as if to reassure them that I was normal, even though I was spending six hours a week carving up a corpse. Sometimes I told of the moment when I turned around and saw a classmate, the sort of woman who had a mug decorated with puffy paint, tiptoeing on a stool, cheerfully hammering a chisel into a woman's backbone, splinters flying through the air. I told this story as if to distance myself from it, but my kinship was undeniable. After all, hadn't I just as eagerly disassembled a man's rib cage with a pair of bolt cutters? Even working on the dead, with their faces covered, their names a mystery, you find that their humanity pops up at you—in opening my cadaver's stomach, I found two undigested morphine pills, meaning that he had died in pain, perhaps alone and fumbling with the cap of a pill bottle.

Of course, the cadavers, in life, donated themselves freely to this fate, and the language surrounding the bodies in front of us soon changed to reflect that fact. We were instructed to no longer call them "cadavers"; "donors" was the preferred term. And yes, the transgressive element of dissection had certainly decreased from the bad old days. (Students no longer had to bring their own bodies, for starters, as they did in the nineteenth century. And medical schools had discontinued their support of the practice of robbing graves to procure cadavers—that looting itself a vast improvement over murder, a means once common enough to warrant its own verb: *burke*, which the OED defines as "to kill secretly by suffocation or strangulation, or for the purpose of selling the victim's body for dissection.") Yet the best-informed people—doctors—almost never donated their bodies. How informed were the donors, then? As one anatomy professor put it to me, "You wouldn't tell a patient the gory details of a surgery if that would make them not consent."

Even if donors were informed enough—and they might well have been, notwithstanding one anatomy professor's hedging—it wasn't so much the thought of being dissected that galled. It was the thought of your mother, your father, your grandparents being hacked to pieces by wisecracking twenty-two-year-old medical students. Every time I read the pre-lab and saw a term like "bone saw," I wondered if this would be the session in which I finally vomited. Yet I was rarely troubled in lab, even when I found that the "bone saw" in question was nothing more than a common, rusty wood saw. The closest I ever came to vomiting was nowhere near the lab but on a visit to my grandmother's grave in New York, on the twentieth anniversary of her death. I found myself doubled over, almost crying, and apologizing— not to my cadaver but to my cadaver's grandchildren. In the midst of our lab, in fact, a son requested his mother's half-dissected body back. Yes, she had consented, but he couldn't live with that. I knew I'd do the same. (The remains were returned.)

In anatomy lab, we objectified the dead, literally reducing them to organs, tissues, nerves, muscles. On that first day, you simply could not deny the humanity of the corpse. But by the time you'd skinned the limbs, sliced through inconvenient muscles, pulled out the lungs, cut open the heart, and removed a lobe of the liver, it was hard to recognize this pile of tissue as human. Anatomy lab, in the end, becomes less a violation of the sacred and more something that interferes with happy hour, and that realization discomfits. In our rare reflective moments, we were all silently apologizing to our cadavers, not because we sensed the transgression but because we did not.

It was not a simple evil, however. All of medicine, not just cadaver dissection, trespasses into sacred spheres. Doctors invade the body in every way imaginable. They see people at their most vulnerable, their most scared, their most private. They escort them into the world, and then back out. Seeing the body as matter and mechanism is the flip side to easing the most profound human suffering. By the same token, the most profound human suffering becomes a mere pedagogical tool. Anatomy professors are perhaps the extreme end of this relationship, yet their kinship to the cadavers remains. Early on, when I made a long, quick cut through my donor's diaphragm in order to ease finding the splenic artery, our proctor was both livid and horrified. Not because I had destroyed an important structure or misunderstood a key concept or ruined a future dissection but because I had seemed so cavalier about it. The look on his face, his inability to vocalize his sadness, taught me more about medicine than any lecture I would ever attend. When I explained that another anatomy professor had told me to make the cut, our proctor's sadness turned to rage, and suddenly red-faced professors were being dragged into the hallway.

Other times, the kinship was much simpler. Once, while showing us the ruins of our donor's pancreatic cancer, the professor asked, "How old is this fellow?"

"Seventy-four," we replied.

"That's my age," he said, set down the probe, and walked away.

• • •

Medical school sharpened my understanding of the relationship between meaning, life, and death. I saw the human relationality I had written about as an undergraduate realized in the doctor-patient relationship. As medical students, we were confronted by death, suffering, and the work entailed in patient care, while being simultaneously shielded from the real brunt of responsibility, though we could spot its specter. Med students spend the first two years in classrooms, socializing, studying, and reading; it was easy to treat the work as a mere extension of undergraduate studies. But my girlfriend, Lucy, whom I met in the first year of medical school (and who would later become my wife), understood the subtext of the academics. Her capacity to love was barely finite, and a lesson to me. One night on the sofa in my apartment, while studying the reams of wavy lines that make up EKGs, she puzzled over, then correctly identified, a fatal arrhythmia. All at once, it dawned on her and she began to cry: wherever this "practice EKG" had come from, the patient had not survived. The squiggly lines on that page were more than just lines; they were ventricular fibrillation deteriorating to asystole, and they could bring you to tears.

Lucy and I attended the Yale School of Medicine when Shep Nuland still lectured there, but I knew him only in my capacity as a reader. Nuland was a renowned surgeon-philosopher whose seminal book about mortality, *How We Die*, had come out when I was in high school but made it into my hands only in medical school. Few books I had read so directly and wholly addressed that fundamental fact of existence: all organisms, whether goldfish or grandchild, die. I pored over it in my room at night, and remember in particular his description of his grandmother's illness, and how that one passage so perfectly illuminated the ways in which the personal, medical, and spiritual all intermingled. Nuland recalled how, as a child, he would play a game in which, using his finger, he indented his grandmother's skin to see how long it took to resume its shape—a part of the aging process that, along with her newfound shortness of breath, showed her "gradual slide into congestive heart failure . . . the significant decline in the amount of oxygen that aged blood is capable of taking up from the aged tissues of the aged lung." But "what was most evident," he continued, "was the slow drawing away from life. . . . By the time Bubbeh stopped praying, she had stopped virtually everything else as well." With her fatal stroke, Nuland remembered Sir Thomas Browne's *Religio Medici*: "With what strife and pains we come into the world we know not, but 'tis commonly no easy matter to get out of it."

I had spent so much time studying literature at Stanford and the history of medicine at Cambridge, in an attempt to better understand the particularities of death, only to come away feeling like they were still unknowable to me. Descriptions like Nuland's convinced me that such things could be known only face-to-face. I was pursuing medicine to bear witness to the twinned mysteries of death, its experiential and biological manifestations: at once deeply personal and utterly impersonal.

I remember Nuland, in the opening chapters of *How We Die*, writing about being a young medical student alone in the OR with a patient whose heart had stopped. In an act of desperation, he cut open the patient's chest and tried to pump his heart manually, tried to literally squeeze the life back into him. The patient died, and Nuland was found by his supervisor, covered in blood and failure.

Medical school had changed by the time I got there,

to the point where such a scene was simply unthinkable: as medical students, we were barely allowed to touch patients, let alone open their chests. What had not changed, though, was the heroic spirit of responsibility amid blood and failure. This struck me as the true image of a doctor.

The first birth I witnessed was also the first death.

I had recently taken Step 1 of my medical boards, wrapping up two years of intensive study buried in books, deep in libraries, poring over lecture notes in coffee shops, reviewing hand-made flash cards while lying in bed. The next two years, then, I would spend in the hospital and clinic, finally putting that theoretical knowledge to use to relieve concrete suffering, with patients, not abstractions, as my primary focus. I started in ob-gyn, working the graveyard shift in the labor and delivery ward.

Walking into the building as the sun descended, I tried to recall the stages of labor, the corresponding dilation of the cervix, the names of the "stations" that indicated the baby's descent—anything that might prove helpful when the time came. As a medical student, my task was to learn by observation and avoid getting in the way. Residents, who had finished medical school and were now completing training in a chosen specialty, and nurses, with their years of clinical experience, would serve as my primary instructors. But the fear still lurked—I could feel its fluttering—that through accident or expectation, I'd be called on to deliver a child by myself, and fail.

I made my way to the doctors' lounge where I was to meet the resident. I walked in and saw a dark-haired young woman lying on a couch, chomping furiously at a sandwich while watching TV and reading a journal article. I introduced myself.

"Oh, hi," she said. "I'm Melissa. I'll be in here or in the call room if you need me. Probably the best thing for you to do is keep an eye on patient Garcia. She's a twenty-two-year-old, here with preterm labor and twins. Everyone else is pretty standard."

Between bites, Melissa briefed me, a barrage of facts and information: The twins were only twenty-three and a half weeks old; the hope was to keep the pregnancy going until they were more developed, however long that might be; twenty-four weeks was considered the cusp of viability, and every extra day made a difference; the patient was getting various drugs to control her contractions. Melissa's pager went off.

"Okay," she said, swinging her legs off the couch. "I gotta go. You can hang out here, if you like. We have good cable channels. Or you can come with me."

I followed Melissa to the nurses' station. One wall was lined with monitors, displaying wavy telemetry lines.

"What's that?" I asked.

"That's the output of the tocometers and the fetal heart rates. Let me show you the patient. She doesn't speak English. Do you speak Spanish?"

I shook my head. Melissa brought me to the room. It was dark. The mother lay in a bed, resting, quiet, monitor bands wrapped around her belly, tracking her contractions and the twins' heart rates and sending the signal to the screens I'd seen at the nurses' station. The father stood at the bedside holding his wife's hand, worry etched on his brow. Melissa whispered something to them in Spanish, then escorted me out.

For the next several hours, things progressed

smoothly. Melissa slept in the lounge. I tried decoding the indecipherable scribbles in Garcia's chart, which was like reading hieroglyphics, and came away with the knowledge that her first name was Elena, this was her second pregnancy, she had received no prenatal care, and she had no insurance. I wrote down the names of the drugs she was getting and made a note to look them up later. I read a little about premature labor in a textbook I found in the doctors' lounge. Preemies, if they survived, apparently incurred high rates of brain hemorrhages and cerebral palsy. Then again, my older brother, Suman, had been born almost eight weeks premature, three decades earlier, and he was now a practicing neurologist. I walked over to the nurse and asked her to teach me how to read those little squiggles on the monitor, which were no clearer to me than the doctors' handwriting but could apparently foretell calm or disaster. She nodded and began talking me through reading a contraction and the fetal hearts' reaction to it, the way, if you looked closely, you could see—

She stopped. Worry flashed across her face. Without a word, she got up and ran into Elena's room, then burst back out, grabbed the phone, and paged Melissa. A minute later, Melissa arrived, bleary-eyed, glanced at the strips, and rushed into the patient's room, with me trailing behind. She flipped open her cellphone and called the attending, rapidly talking in a jargon I only partially understood. The twins were in distress, I gathered, and their only shot at survival was an emergency C-section.

I was carried along with the commotion into the operating room. They got Elena supine on the table, drugs running into her veins. A nurse frantically painted the woman's swollen abdomen with an antiseptic solution, while the attending, the resident, and I splashed alcohol cleanser on our hands and forearms. I mimicked their urgent strokes, standing silently as they cursed under their breath. The anesthesiologists intubated the patient while the senior surgeon, the attending, fidgeted.

"C'mon," he said. "We don't have a lot of time. We need to move faster!"

I was standing next to the attending as he sliced open the woman's belly, making a single long curvilinear incision beneath her belly button, just below the apex of her protuberant womb. I tried to follow every movement, digging in my brain for textbook anatomical sketches. The skin slid apart at the scalpel's touch. He sliced confidently through the tough white rectus fascia covering the muscle, then split the fascia and the underlying muscle with his hands, revealing the first glimpse of the melon-like uterus. He sliced that open as well, and a small face appeared, then disappeared amid the blood. In plunged the doctor's hands, pulling out one, then two purple babies, barely moving, eyes fused shut, like tiny birds fallen too soon from a nest. With their bones visible through translucent skin, they looked more like the preparatory sketches of children than children themselves. Too small to cradle, not much bigger than the surgeon's hands, they were rapidly passed to the waiting neonatal intensivists, who rushed them to the neonatal ICU.

With the immediate danger averted, the pace of the operation slowed, frenzy turning to something resembling calm. The odor of burnt flesh wafted up as the cautery arrested little spurts of blood. The uterus was sutured back together, the stitches like a row of teeth, biting closed the open wound.

"Professor, do you want the peritoneum closed?" Melissa asked. "I read recently that it doesn't need to be."

"Let no man put asunder what God has joined," the

attending said. "At least, no more than temporarily. I like to leave things the way I found them—let's sew it back up."

The peritoneum is a membrane that surrounds the abdominal cavity. Somehow I had completely missed its opening, and I couldn't see it at all now. To me, the wound looked like a mass of disorganized tissue, yet to the surgeons it had an appreciable order, like a block of marble to a sculptor.

Melissa called for the peritoneal stitch, reached her forceps into the wound, and pulled up a transparent layer of tissue between the muscle and the uterus. Suddenly the peritoneum, and the gaping hole in it, was clear. She sewed it closed and moved on to the muscle and fascia, putting them back together with a large needle and a few big looping stitches. The attending left, and finally the skin was sutured together. Melissa asked me if I wanted to place the last two stitches.

My hands shook as I passed the needle through the subcutaneous tissue. As I tightened down the suture, I saw that the needle was slightly bent. The skin had come together lopsided, a glob of fat poking through.

Melissa sighed. "That's uneven," she said. "You have

to *just* catch the dermal layer—you see this thin white stripe?"

I did. Not only would my mind have to be trained, my eyes would, too.

"Scissors!" Melissa cut out my amateur knots, resutured the wound, applied the dressing, and the patient was taken to recovery.

As Melissa had told me earlier, twenty-four weeks in utero was considered the edge of viability. The twins had lasted twenty-three weeks and six days. Their organs were present, but perhaps not yet ready for the responsibility of sustaining life. They were owed nearly four more months of protected development in the womb, where oxygenated blood and nutrients came to them through the umbilical cord. Now oxygen would have to come through the lungs, and the lungs were not capable of the complex expansion and gas transfer that was respiration. I went to see them in the NICU, each twin encased in a clear plastic incubator, dwarfed by large, beeping machines, barely visible amid the tangle of wires and tubes. The incubator had small side ports through which the parents could strain to reach and gently stroke a leg or arm, providing vital human contact.

The sun was up, my shift over. I was sent home, the image of the twins being extracted from the uterus interrupting my sleep. Like a premature lung, I felt unready for the responsibility of sustaining life.

When I returned to work that night, I was assigned to a new mother. No one anticipated problems with this pregnancy. Things were as routine as possible; today was even her actual due date. Along with the nurse, I followed the mother's steady progress, contractions racking her body with increasing regularity. The nurse reported the dilation of the cervix, from three centimeters to five to ten.

"Okay, it's time to push now," the nurse said.

Turning to me, she said, "Don't worry—we'll page you when the delivery is close."

I found Melissa in the doctors' lounge. After some time, the OB team was called into the room: delivery was near. Outside the door, Melissa handed me a gown, gloves, and a pair of long boot covers.

"It gets messy," she said.

We entered the room. I stood awkwardly off to the side until Melissa pushed me to the front, between the patient's legs, just in front of the attending.

"Push!" the nurse encouraged. "Now again: just like that, only without the screaming."

The screaming didn't stop, and was soon accompanied by a gush of blood and other fluids. The neatness of medical diagrams did nothing to represent Nature, red not only in tooth and claw but in birth as well. (An Anne Geddes photo this was not.) It was becoming clear that learning to be a doctor in practice was going to be a very different education from being a medical student in the classroom. Reading books and answering multiple-choice questions bore little resemblance to taking action, with its concomitant responsibility. Knowing you need to be judicious when pulling on the head to facilitate delivery of the shoulder is not the same as doing it. What if I pulled too hard? (*Irreversible nerve injury*, my brain shouted.) The head appeared with each push and then retracted with each break, three steps forward, two steps back. I waited. The human brain has rendered the organism's most basic task, reproduction, a treacherous affair. That same brain made things like labor and delivery units, cardiotocometers, epidurals, and emergency C-sections both possible *and* necessary.

I stood still, unsure when to act or what to do. The

attending's voice guided my hands to the emerging head, and on the next push, I gently guided the baby's shoulders as she came out. She was large, plump, and wet, easily three times the size of the birdlike creatures from the previous night. Melissa clamped the cord, and I cut it. The child's eyes opened and she began to cry. I held the baby a moment longer, feeling her weight and substance, then passed her to the nurse, who brought her to the mother.

I walked out to the waiting room to inform the extended family of the happy news. The dozen or so family members gathered there leapt up to celebrate, a riot of handshakes and hugs. I was a prophet returning from the mountaintop with news of a joyous new covenant! All the messiness of the birth disappeared; here I had just been holding the newest member of this family, this man's niece, this girl's cousin.

Returning to the ward, ebullient, I ran into Melissa.

"Hey, do you know how last night's twins are doing?" I asked.

She darkened. Baby A died yesterday afternoon; Baby B managed to live not quite twenty-four hours, then passed away around the time I was delivering the new baby. In that moment, I could only think of Samuel Beckett, the metaphors that, in those twins, reached their terminal limit: "One day we were born, one day we shall die, the same day, the same second.... Birth astride of a grave, the light gleams an instant, then it's night once more." I had stood next to "the grave digger" with his "forceps." What had these lives amounted to?

"You think *that's* bad?" she continued. "Most mothers with stillborns still have to go through labor and deliver. Can you imagine? At least these guys had a chance."

A match flickers but does not light. The mother's wailing in room 543, the searing red rims of the father's lower eyelids, tears silently streaking his face: this flip side of joy, the unbearable, unjust, unexpected presence of death ... What possible sense could be made, what words were there for comfort?

"Was it the right choice, to do an emergency C-section?" I asked.

"No question," she said. "It was the only shot they had."

"What happens if you don't?"

"Probably, they die. Abnormal fetal heart tracings show when the fetal blood is turning acidemic; the cord is compromised somehow, or something else seriously bad is happening."

"But how do you know when the tracing looks bad enough? Which is worse, being born too early or waiting too long to deliver?"

"Judgment call."

What a call to make. In my life, had I ever made a decision harder than choosing between a French dip and a Reuben? How could I ever learn to make, and live with, such judgment calls? I still had a lot of practical medicine to learn, but would knowledge alone be enough, with life and death hanging in the balance? Surely intelligence wasn't enough; moral clarity was needed as well. Somehow, I had to believe, I would gain not only knowledge but wisdom, too. After all, when I had walked into the hospital just one day before, birth and death had been merely abstract concepts. Now I had seen them both up close. Maybe Beckett's Pozzo is right. Maybe life *is* merely an "instant," too brief to consider. But my focus would have to be on my imminent role, intimately involved with the when and how of death—the grave digger with the forceps.

Not long after, my ob-gyn rotation ended, and it was

immediately on to surgical oncology. Mari, a fellow med student, and I would rotate together. A few weeks in, after a sleepless night, she was assigned to assist in a Whipple, a complex operation that involves rearranging most abdominal organs in an attempt to resect pancreatic cancer, an operation in which a medical student typically stands still—or, at best, retracts—for up to nine hours straight. It's considered the plum operation to be selected to help with, because of its extreme complexity—only chief residents are allowed to actively participate. But it is grueling, the ultimate test of a general surgeon's skill. Fifteen minutes after the operation started, I saw Mari in the hallway, crying. The surgeon always begins a Whipple by inserting a small camera through a tiny incision to look for metastases, as widespread cancer renders the operation useless and causes its cancellation. Standing there, waiting in the OR with a nine-hour surgery stretching out before her, Mari had a whisper of a thought: *I'm so tired—please God, let there be mets.* There were. The patient was sewn back up, the procedure called off. First came relief, then a gnawing, deepening shame. Mari burst out of the OR, where, needing a confessor, she saw me, and I became one.

pay, work environment, hours. But that's the point. Putting lifestyle first is how you find a job—not a calling.)

As for me, I would choose neurosurgery as my specialty. The choice, which I had been contemplating for some time, was cemented one night in a room just off the OR, when I listened in quiet awe as a pediatric neurosurgeon sat down with the parents of a child with a large brain tumor who had come in that night complaining of headaches. He not only delivered the clinical facts but addressed the human facts as well, acknowledging the tragedy of the situation and providing guidance. As it happened, the child's mother was a radiologist. The tumor looked malignant—the mother had already studied the scans, and now she sat in a plastic chair, under fluorescent light, devastated.

"Now, Claire," the surgeon began, softly.

"Is it as bad as it looks?" the mother interrupted. "Do you think it's cancer?"

"I don't know. What I *do* know—and I know you know these things, too—is that your life is about to—it already has changed. This is going to be a long haul, you understand? You have got to be there for each other, but you also have to get your rest when you need it. This kind of illness can either bring you together, or it can tear you apart. Now more than ever, you have to be there for each other. I don't want either of you staying up all night at the bedside or never leaving the hospital. Okay?"

He went on to describe the planned operation, the likely outcomes and possibilities, what decisions needed to be made now, what decisions they should start thinking about but didn't need to decide on immediately, and what sorts of decisions they should not worry about at all yet. By the end of the conversation, the family was not at ease, but they seemed able to face the future. I had watched the parents' faces—at first wan, dull, almost otherworldly—sharpen and focus. And as I sat there, I realized that the questions intersecting life, death, and meaning, questions that all people face at some point, usually arise in a medical context. In the actual situations where one encounters these questions, it becomes a necessarily philosophical and biological exercise. Humans are organisms, subject to physical laws, including, alas, the one that says entropy always increases. Diseases are molecules misbehaving; the basic requirement of life is metabolism, and death its cessation.

While all doctors treat diseases, neurosurgeons work in the crucible of identity: every operation on the brain is, by necessity, a manipulation of the substance of our selves, and every conversation with a patient undergoing brain surgery cannot help but confront this fact. In addition, to the patient and family, the brain surgery is usually the most dramatic event they have ever faced and, as such, has the impact of any major life event. At those critical junctures, the question is not simply whether to live or die but what kind of life is worth living. Would you trade your ability—or your mother's—to talk for a few extra months of mute life? The expansion of your visual blind spot in exchange for eliminating the small possibility of a fatal brain hemorrhage? Your right hand's function to stop seizures? How much neurologic suffering would you let your child endure before saying that death is preferable? Because the brain mediates our experience of the world, any neurosurgical problem forces a patient and family, ideally with a doctor as a guide, to answer this question: What makes life meaningful enough to go on living?

I was compelled by neurosurgery, with its unforgiving call to perfection; like the ancient Greek concept *arete*, I thought, virtue required moral, emotional, mental, and physical excellence. Neurosurgery seemed to present the most challenging and direct confrontation with meaning, identity, and death. Concomitant with the enormous responsibilities they shouldered, neurosurgeons were also masters of many fields: neurosurgery, ICU medicine, neurology, radiology. Not only would I have to train my mind and hands, I realized; I'd have to train my eyes, and perhaps other organs as well. The idea was overwhelming and intoxicating: perhaps I, too, could join the ranks of these polymaths who strode into the densest thicket of emotional, scientific, and spiritual problems and found, or carved, ways out.

After medical school, Lucy and I, newly married, headed to California to begin our residencies, me at Stanford, Lucy just up the road at UCSF. Medical school was officially behind us—now real responsibility lay in wait. In short order, I made several close friends in the hospital, in particular Victoria, my co-resident, and Jeff, a general surgery resident a few years senior to us. Over the next seven years of training, we would grow from bearing witness to medical dramas to becoming leading actors in them.

As an intern in the first year of residency, one is little more than a paper pusher against a backdrop of life and death—though, even then, the workload is enormous. My first day in the hospital, the chief resident said to me, "Neurosurgery residents aren't just the best surgeons—we're the best *doctors* in the hospital. That's your goal. Make us proud." The chairman, passing through the ward: "Always eat with your left hand. You've got to learn to be ambidextrous." One of the senior residents: "Just a heads-up—the chief is going through a divorce, so he's really throwing himself into his work right now. Don't make small talk with him." The outgoing intern who was supposed to orient me but instead just handed me a list of forty-three patients: "The only thing I have to tell you is: they can always hurt you more, but they can't stop the clock." And then he walked away.

I didn't leave the hospital for the first two days, but before long, the impossible-seeming, day-killing mounds of paperwork were only an hour's work. Still, when you work in a hospital, the papers you file aren't just papers: they are fragments of narratives filled with risks and triumphs. An eight-year-old named Matthew, for example, came in one day complaining of headaches only to learn that he had a tumor abutting his hypothalamus. The hypothalamus regulates our basic drives: sleep, hunger, thirst, sex. Leaving any tumor behind would subject Matthew to a life of radiation, further surgeries, brain catheters . . . in short, it would consume his childhood. Complete removal could prevent that, but at the risk of damaging his hypothalamus, rendering him a slave to his appetites. The surgeon got to work, passed a small endoscope through Matthew's nose, and drilled off the floor of his skull. Once inside, he saw a clear plane and removed the tumor. A few days later, Matthew was bopping around the ward, sneaking candies from the nurses, ready to go home. That night, I happily filled out the endless pages of his discharge paperwork.

I lost my first patient on a Tuesday.

She was an eighty-two-year-old woman, small and trim, the healthiest person on the general surgery service, where I spent a month as an intern. (At her autopsy, the pathologist would be shocked to learn her age: "She has the organs of a fifty-year-old!") She had been admitted for constipation from a mild bowel obstruction. After six days of hoping her bowels would untangle themselves, we did a minor operation to help sort things out. Around eight P.M. Monday night, I stopped by to check on her, and she was alert, doing fine. As we talked, I pulled from my pocket my list of the day's work and crossed off the last item (post-op check, Mrs. Harvey). It was time to go home and get some rest.

Sometime after midnight, the phone rang. The patient was crashing. With the complacency of bureaucratic work suddenly torn away, I sat up in bed and spat out orders: "One liter bolus of LR, EKG, chest X-ray, stat—I'm on my way in." I called my chief, and she told me to add labs and to call her back when I had a better sense of things. I sped to the hospital and found Mrs. Harvey struggling for air, her heart racing, her blood pressure collapsing. She wasn't getting better no matter what I did; and as I was the only general surgery intern on call, my pager was buzzing relentlessly, with calls I could dispense with (patients needing sleep medication) and ones I couldn't (a rupturing aortic aneurysm in the ER). I was drowning, out of my depth, pulled in a thousand directions, and Mrs. Harvey was still not improving. I arranged a transfer to the ICU, where we blasted her with drugs and fluids to keep her from dying, and I spent the next few hours running between my patient threatening to die in the ER and my patient actively dying in the ICU. By 5:45 A.M., the patient in the ER was on his way to the OR, and Mrs. Harvey was relatively stable. She'd needed twelve liters of fluid, two units of blood, a ventilator, and three different pressors to stay alive.

When I finally left the hospital, at five P.M. on Tuesday evening, Mrs. Harvey wasn't getting better—or worse. At seven P.M., the phone rang: Mrs. Harvey had coded, and the ICU team was attempting CPR. I raced back to the hospital, and once again, she pulled through. Barely. This time, instead of going home, I grabbed dinner near the hospital, just in case.

At eight P.M., my phone rang: Mrs. Harvey had died.

I went home to sleep.

I was somewhere between angry and sad. For whatever reason, Mrs. Harvey had burst through the layers of paperwork to become my patient. The next day, I attended her autopsy, watched the pathologists open her up and remove her organs. I inspected them myself, ran my hands over them, checked the knots I had tied in her intestines. From that point on, I resolved to treat all my paperwork as patients, and not vice versa.

In that first year, I would glimpse my share of death. I sometimes saw it while peeking around corners, other times while feeling embarrassed to be caught in the same room. Here were a few of the people I saw die:

1. An alcoholic, his blood no longer able to clot, who bled to death into his joints and under his skin. Every day, the bruises would spread. Before he became delirious, he looked up at me and said, "It's not fair—I've been diluting my drinks with water."

2. A pathologist, dying of pneumonia, wheezing her death rattle before heading down to be autopsied—her final trip to the pathology lab, where she had spent so many years of her life.

3. A man who'd had a minor neurosurgical procedure to treat lightning bolts of pain that were shooting through his face: a tiny drop of liquid cement had been placed on the suspected nerve to

keep a vein from pressing on it. A week later, he developed massive headaches. Nearly every test was run, but no diagnosis was ever identified.

4. Dozens of cases of head trauma: suicides, gunshots, bar fights, motorcycle accidents, car crashes. A moose attack.

At moments, the weight of it all became palpable. It was in the air, the stress and misery. Normally, you breathed it in, without noticing it. But some days, like a humid muggy day, it had a suffocating weight of its own. Some days, this is how it felt when I was in the hospital: trapped in an endless jungle summer, wet with sweat, the rain of tears of the families of the dying pouring down.

In the second year of training, you're the first to arrive in an emergency. Some patients you can't save. Others you can: the first time I rushed a comatose patient from the ER to the OR, drained the blood from his skull, and then watched him wake up, start talking to his family, and complain about the incision on his head, I got lost in a euphoric daze, promenading around the hospital at two A.M. until I had no sense of where I was. It took me forty-five minutes to find my way back out.

The schedule took a toll. As residents, we were working as much as one hundred hours a week; though regulations officially capped our hours at eighty-eight, there was always more work to be done. My eyes watered, my head throbbed, I downed energy drinks at two A.M. At work, I could keep it together, but as soon as I walked out of the hospital, the exhaustion would hit me. I staggered through the parking lot, often napping in my car before driving the fifteen minutes home to bed.

Not all residents could stand the pressure. One was simply unable to accept blame or responsibility. He was a talented surgeon, but he could not admit when he'd made a mistake. I sat with him one day in the lounge as he begged me to help him save his career.

"All you have to do," I said, "is look me in the eye and say, 'I'm sorry. What happened was my fault, and I won't let it happen again.'"

"But it was the nurse who—"

"No. You have to be able to say it and mean it. Try again."

79

"But—"

"No. *Say* it."

This went on for an hour before I knew he was doomed.

The stress drove another resident out of the field entirely; she elected to leave for a less taxing job in consulting.

Others would pay even higher prices.

As my skills increased, so too did my responsibility. Learning to judge whose lives could be saved, whose couldn't be, and whose *shouldn't* be requires an unattainable prognostic ability. I made mistakes. Rushing a patient to the OR to save only enough brain that his heart beats but he can never speak, he eats through a tube, and he is condemned to an existence he would never want . . . I came to see this as a more egregious failure than the patient dying. The twilight existence of unconscious metabolism becomes an unbearable burden, usually left to an institution, where the family, unable to attain closure, visits with increasing rarity, until the inevitable fatal bedsore or pneumonia sets in. Some insist on this life and embrace its possibility, eyes open. But many do not, or cannot, and the neurosurgeon must learn to adjudicate.

I had started in this career, in part, to pursue death: to grasp it, uncloak it, and see it eye-to-eye, unblinking. Neurosurgery attracted me as much for its intertwining of brain and consciousness as for its intertwining of life and death. I had thought that a life spent in the space between the two would grant me not merely a stage for compassionate action but an elevation of my own being: getting as far away from petty materialism, from self-important trivia, getting *right there*, to the heart of the matter, to truly life-and-death decisions and struggles ... surely a kind of transcendence would be found there?

But in residency, something else was gradually unfolding. In the midst of this endless barrage of head injuries, I began to suspect that being so close to the fiery light of such moments only blinded me to their nature, like trying to learn astronomy by staring directly at the sun. I was not yet *with* patients in their pivotal moments, I was merely *at* those pivotal moments. I observed a lot of suffering; worse, I became inured to it. Drowning, even in blood, one adapts, learns to float, to swim, even to enjoy life, bonding with the nurses, doctors, and others who are clinging to the same raft, caught in the same tide.

My fellow resident Jeff and I worked traumas together. When he called me down to the trauma bay because of a concurrent head injury, we were always in sync. He'd assess the abdomen, then ask for my prognosis on a patient's cognitive function. "Well, he could still be a senator," I once replied, "but only from a small state." Jeff laughed, and from that moment on, state population became our barometer for head-injury severity. "Is he a Wyoming or a California?" Jeff would ask, trying to determine how intensive his care plan should be. Or I'd say, "Jeff, I know his blood pressure is labile, but I gotta get him to the OR or he's gonna go from Washington to Idaho—can you get him stabilized?"

In the cafeteria one day, as I was grabbing my typical lunch—a Diet Coke and an ice cream sandwich—my pager announced an incoming major trauma. I ran to the trauma bay, tucking my ice cream sandwich behind a computer just as the paramedics arrived, pushing the gurney, reciting the details: "Twenty-two-year-old male, motorcycle accident, forty miles per hour, possible brain coming out his nose . . ."

I went straight to work, calling for an intubation tray, assessing his other vital functions. Once he was safely intubated, I surveyed his various injuries: the bruised face, the road rash, the dilated pupils. We pumped him full of mannitol to reduce brain swelling and rushed him to the scanner: a shattered skull, heavy diffuse bleeding. In my mind, I was already planning the scalp incision, how I'd drill the bone, evacuate the blood. His blood pressure suddenly dropped. We rushed him back to the trauma bay, and just as the rest of the trauma team arrived, his heart stopped. A whirlwind of activity surrounded him: catheters were slipped into his femoral arteries, tubes shoved deep into his chest, drugs pushed into his IVs, and all the while, fists pounded on his heart to keep the blood flowing. After thirty minutes, we let him finish dying. With that kind of head injury, we all murmured in agreement, death was to be preferred.

I slipped out of the trauma bay just as the family was brought in to view the body. Then I remembered: my Diet Coke, my ice cream sandwich . . . and the sweltering heat of the trauma bay. With one of the ER residents covering for me, I slipped back in, ghostlike, to save the ice cream sandwich in front of the corpse of the son I could not.

Thirty minutes in the freezer resuscitated the sandwich. *Pretty tasty*, I thought, picking chocolate chips out of my teeth as the family said its last goodbyes. I wondered if, in my brief time as a physician, I had made more moral slides than strides.

A few days later, I heard that Laurie, a friend from medical school, had been hit by a car and that a neurosurgeon had performed an operation to try to save her. She'd coded, was revived, and then died the following day. I didn't want to know more. The days when someone was simply "killed in a car accident" were long gone. Now those words opened a Pandora's box, out of which emerged all the images: the roll of the gurney, the blood on the trauma bay floor, the tube shoved down her throat, the pounding on her chest. I could see hands, my hands, shaving Laurie's scalp, the scalpel cutting open her head, could hear the frenzy of the drill and smell the burning bone, its dust whirling, the crack as I pried off a section of her skull. Her hair half shaven, her head deformed. She failed to resemble herself at all; she became a stranger to her friends and family. Maybe there were chest tubes, and a leg was in traction . . .

I didn't ask for details. I already had too many.

In that moment, all my occasions of failed empathy came rushing back to me: the times I had pushed discharge over patient worries, ignored patients' pain when other demands pressed. The people whose suffering I saw, noted, and neatly packaged into various diagnoses, the significance of which I failed to recognize—they all returned, vengeful, angry, and inexorable.

I feared I was on the way to becoming Tolstoy's stereotype of a doctor, preoccupied with empty formalism, focused on the rote treatment of disease—and utterly missing the larger human significance. ("Doctors came to see her singly and in consultation, talked much in French, German, and Latin, blamed one another, and prescribed a great variety of medicines for all the diseases known to them, but the simple idea never occurred to any of them that they could not know the disease Natasha was suffering from.") A mother came to me, newly diagnosed with brain cancer. She was confused, scared, overcome by uncertainty. I was exhausted, disconnected. I rushed through her questions, assured her that surgery would be a success, and assured myself that there wasn't enough time to answer her questions fairly. *But why didn't I make the time?* A truculent vet refused the advice and coaxing of doctors, nurses, and physical therapists for weeks; as a result, his back wound broke down, just as we had warned him it would. Called out of the OR, I stitched the dehiscent wound as he yelped in pain, telling myself he'd had it coming.

Nobody has it coming.

I took meager solace in knowing that William Carlos Williams and Richard Selzer had confessed to doing worse, and I swore to do better. Amid the tragedies and failures, I feared I was losing sight of the singular importance of human relationships, not between patients and their families but between doctor and patient. Technical excellence was not enough. As a resident, my highest ideal was not saving lives—everyone dies eventually—but guiding a patient or family to an understanding of death or illness. When a patient comes in with a fatal head bleed, that first conversation with a neurosurgeon may forever color how the family remembers the death, from a peaceful letting go ("Maybe it was his time") to an open sore of regret ("Those doctors didn't listen! They didn't even *try* to save him!"). When there's no place for the scalpel, words are the surgeon's only tool.

For amid that unique suffering invoked by severe brain damage, the suffering often felt more by families than by patients, it is not merely the physicians who do not see the full significance. The families who gather around their beloved—their beloved whose sheared heads contained battered brains—do not usually recognize the full significance, either. They see the past, the accumulation of memories, the freshly felt love, all represented by the body before them. I see the possible futures, the breathing machines connected through a surgical opening in the neck, the pasty liquid dripping in through a hole in the belly, the possible long, painful, and only partial recovery—or, sometimes more likely, no return at all of the person they remember. In these moments, I acted not, as I most often did, as death's enemy, but as its ambassador. I had to help those families understand that the person they knew—the full, vital independent human—now lived only in the past and that I needed their input to understand what sort of future he or she would want: an easy death or to be strung between bags of fluids going in, others coming out, to persist despite being unable to struggle.

Had I been more religious in my youth, I might have become a pastor, for it was the pastoral role I'd sought.

With my renewed focus, informed consent—the ritual by which a patient signs a piece of paper, authorizing surgery—became not a juridical exercise in naming all the risks as quickly as possible, like the voiceover in an ad for a new pharmaceutical, but an opportunity to forge a covenant with a suffering compatriot: *Here we are together, and here are the ways through—I promise to guide you, as best as I can, to the other side.*

By this point in my residency, I was more efficient and experienced. I could finally breathe a little, no longer trying to hang on for my own dear life. I was now accepting full responsibility for my patients' well-being.

My thoughts turned to my father. As medical students, Lucy and I had attended his hospital rounds in Kingman, watching as he brought comfort and levity to his patients. To one woman, who was recovering from a cardiac procedure: "Are you hungry? What can I get you to eat?"

"Anything," she said. "I'm starving."

"Well, how about lobster and steak?" He picked up the phone and called the nursing station. "My patient needs lobster and steak—right away!" Turning back to her, he said, with a smile: "It's on the way, but it may look more like a turkey sandwich."

The easy human connections he formed, the trust he instilled in his patients, were an inspiration to me.

A thirty-five-year-old sat in her ICU bed, a sheen of terror on her face. She had been shopping for her sister's birthday when she'd had a seizure. A scan showed that a benign brain tumor was pressing on her right frontal lobe. In terms of operative risk, it was the best kind of tumor to have, and the best place to have it; surgery would almost certainly eliminate her seizures. The alternative was a lifetime on toxic antiseizure medications. But I could see that the idea of brain surgery terrified her, more than most. She was lonesome and in a strange place, having been swept out of the familiar hubbub of a shopping mall and into the alien beeps and alarms and antiseptic smells of an ICU. She would likely refuse surgery if I launched into a detached spiel detailing all the risks and possible complications. I could do so, document her refusal in the chart, consider my duty discharged, and move on to the next task. Instead, with her permission, I gathered her family with her, and together we calmly talked through the options. As we talked, I could see the enormousness of the choice she faced dwindle into a difficult but understandable decision. I had met her in a space where she was a person, instead of a problem to be solved. She chose surgery. The operation went smoothly. She went home two days later, and never seized again.

Any major illness transforms a patient's—really, an entire family's—life. But brain diseases have the additional strangeness of the esoteric. A son's death already defies the parents' ordered universe; how much more incomprehensible is it when the patient is brain-dead, his body warm, his heart still beating? The root of *disaster* means a star coming apart, and no image expresses better the look in a patient's eyes when hearing a neurosurgeon's diagnosis. Sometimes the news so shocks the mind that the brain suffers an electrical short. This phenomenon is known as a "psychogenic" syndrome, a severe version of the swoon some experience after hearing bad news. When my mother, alone at college, heard that her father, who had championed her right to an education in rural 1960s India, had finally died after a long hospitalization, she had a psychogenic seizure—which continued until she returned home to attend the funeral. One of my patients, upon being diagnosed with brain cancer, fell suddenly into a coma. I ordered a battery of labs, scans, and EEGs, searching for a cause, without result. The definitive test was the simplest: I raised the patient's arm above his face and let go. A patient in a psychogenic coma retains just enough volition to avoid hitting himself. The treatment consists in speaking reassuringly, until your words connect and the patient awakens.

Cancer of the brain comes in two varieties: primary cancers, which are born in the brain, and metastases, which emigrate from somewhere else in the body, most commonly from the lungs. Surgery does not cure the disease, but it does prolong life; for most people, cancer in the brain suggests death within a year, maybe two. Mrs. Lee was in her late fifties, with pale green eyes, and could see the vastness of the chasm between the life she'd had last week and the one she was about to enter. She and her husband didn't seem ready to hear *brain cancer*—is anyone?—so I began a couple steps back. "The MRI shows a mass in your brain, which is causing your symptoms."

Silence.

"Do you want to see the MRI?"

"Yes."

I brought up the images on the bedside computer, pointing out her nose, eyes, and ears to orient her. Then I scrolled up to the tumor, a lumpy white ring surrounding a black necrotic core.

"What's that?" she asked.

Could be anything. Maybe an infection. We won't know till after surgery.

My inclination to dodge the question still persisted, to let their obvious worries float in their heads, unpinned.

"We can't be sure until after surgery," I began, "but it looks very much like a brain tumor."

"Is it cancer?"

"Again, we won't know for certain until it is removed

and examined by our pathologists, but, if I had to guess, I would say yes."

Based on the scan, there was no doubt in my mind that this was glioblastoma—an aggressive brain cancer, the worst kind. Yet I proceeded softly, taking my cues from Mrs. Lee and her husband. Having introduced the possibility of brain cancer, I doubted they would recall much else. A tureen of tragedy was best allotted by the spoonful. Only a few patients demanded the whole at once; most needed time to digest. They didn't ask about prognosis—unlike in trauma, where you have only about ten minutes to explain and make a major decision, here I could let things settle. I discussed in detail what to expect over the next couple of days: what the surgery entailed; how we'd shave only a small strip of her hair to keep it cosmetically appealing; how her arm would likely get a little weaker afterward but then stronger again; that if all went well, she'd be out of the hospital in three days; that this was just the first step in a marathon; that getting rest was important; and that I didn't expect them to retain anything I had just said and we'd go over everything again.

After surgery, we talked again, this time discussing chemo, radiation, and prognosis. By this point, I had learned a couple of basic rules. First, detailed statistics are for research halls, not hospital rooms. The standard statistic, the Kaplan-Meier curve, measures the number of patients surviving over time. It is the metric by which we gauge progress, by which we understand the ferocity of a disease. For glioblastoma, the curve drops sharply until only about 5 percent of patients are alive at two years. Second, it is important to be accurate, but you must always leave some room for hope. Rather than saying, "Median survival is eleven months" or "You have a ninety-five percent chance of being dead in two years," I'd say, "Most patients live many months to a couple of years." This was, to me, a more honest description. The problem is that you can't tell an individual patient where she sits on the curve: Will she die in six months or sixty? I came to believe that it is irresponsible to be more precise than you can be accurate. Those apocryphal doctors who gave specific numbers ("The doctor told me I had six months to live"): Who were they, I wondered, and who taught them statistics?

Patients, when hearing the news, mostly remain mute. (One of the early meanings of *patient*, after all, is "one who endures hardship without complaint.") Whether out of dignity or shock, silence usually reigns, and so holding a patient's hand becomes the mode of communication. A few immediately harden (usually the spouse, rather than the patient): "We're gonna fight and beat this thing, Doc." The armament varies, from prayer to wealth to herbs to stem cells. To me, that hardness always seems brittle, unrealistic optimism the only alternative to crushing despair. In any case, in the immediacy of surgery, a warlike attitude fit. In the OR, the dark gray rotting tumor seemed an invader in the fleshy peach convolutions of the brain, and I felt real anger (*Got you, you fucker*, I muttered). Removing the tumor was satisfying—even though I knew that microscopic cancer cells had already spread throughout that healthy-looking brain. The nearly inevitable recurrence was a problem for another day. A spoonful at a time. Openness to human relationality does not mean revealing grand truths from the apse; it means meeting patients where they are, in the narthex or nave, and bringing them as far as you can.

Yet openness to human relationality also carried a price.

One evening in my third year, I ran into Jeff, my friend in general surgery, a similarly intense and demanding profession. We each noted the other's despondency. "You go first," he said. And I described the death of a child, shot in the head for wearing the wrong color shoes, but he had been so close to making it ... Amid a recent spate of fatal, inoperable brain tumors, my hopes had been pinned on this kid pulling through, and he hadn't. Jeff paused, and I awaited his story. Instead, he laughed, punched me in the arm, and said, "Well, I guess I learned one thing: if I'm ever feeling down about my work, I can always talk to a neurosurgeon to cheer myself up."

Driving home later that night, after gently explaining to a mother that her newborn had been born without a brain and would die shortly, I switched on the radio; NPR was reporting on the continuing drought in California. Suddenly, tears were streaming down my face.

Being *with* patients in these moments certainly had its emotional cost, but it also had its rewards. I don't think I ever spent a minute of any day wondering why I did this work, or whether it was worth it. The call to protect life—and not merely life but another's identity; it is perhaps not too much to say another's soul—was obvious in its sacredness.

Before operating on a patient's brain, I realized, I must first understand his mind: his identity, his values, what makes his life worth living, and what devastation makes it reasonable to let that life end. The cost of my dedication to succeed was high, and the ineluctable failures brought me nearly unbearable guilt. Those burdens are what make medicine holy and wholly impossible: in taking up another's cross, one must sometimes get crushed by the weight.

Midway through residency, time is set aside for additional training. Perhaps unique in medicine, the ethos of neurosurgery—of excellence in all things—maintains that excellence in neurosurgery alone is not enough. In order to carry the field, neurosurgeons must venture forth and excel in other fields as well. Sometimes this is very public, as in the case of the neurosurgeon-journalist Sanjay Gupta, but most often the doctor's focus is on a related field. The most rigorous and prestigious path is that of the neurosurgeon-neuroscientist.

In my fourth year, I began work in a Stanford lab dedicated to basic motor neuroscience and the development of neural prosthetic technology that would allow, say, paralyzed people to mentally control a computer cursor or robot arm. The head of the lab, a professor of electrical engineering and neurobiology, a fellow second-generation Indian, was affectionately called "V" by everyone. V was seven years older than I, but we got on like brothers. His lab had become a world leader in reading out brain signals, but with his blessing I embarked on a project to do the reverse: to write signals *into* the brain. After all, if your robot arm can't *feel* how hard it's grasping a wineglass, you will break a lot of wineglasses. The implications of writing signals into the brain, or "neuromodulation," however, were far more wide-reaching than that: being able to control neural firing would conceivably allow treatment of a host of currently untreatable or intractable neurological and psychiatric diseases, from major depression to Huntington's to schizophrenia to Tourette's to OCD ... the possibilities were limitless. Putting surgery aside now, I set to work learning to apply new techniques in gene therapy in a series of "first of its kind" experiments.

After I'd been there for a year, V and I sat down for one of our weekly meetings. I had grown to love these chats. V was not like other scientists I knew. He was soft-spoken and cared deeply about people and the clinical mission, and he often confessed to me that he wished he'd been a surgeon himself. Science, I had come to learn, is as political, competitive, and fierce a career as you can find, full of the temptation to find easy paths.

One could count on V to always choose the honest (and, often, self-effacing) way forward. While most scientists connived to publish in the most prestigious journals and get their names out there, V maintained that our only obligation was to be authentic to the scientific story and to tell it uncompromisingly. I'd never met someone so successful who was also so committed to goodness. V was an actual paragon.

Instead of smiling as I sat down across from him, he looked pained. He sighed and said, "I need you to wear your doctor hat right now."

"Okay."

"They tell me I have pancreatic cancer."

"V . . . okay. Tell me the story."

He laid out his gradual weight loss, indigestion, and his recent "precautionary" CT scan—a truly nonstandard procedure at this point—which showed a pancreatic mass. We discussed the way forward, the dreaded Whipple operation in his near future ("You are going to feel like a truck hit you," I told him), who the best surgeons were, the impact the illness would have on his wife and children, and how to run the lab during his prolonged absence. Pancreatic cancer has a dismal prognosis, but of course there was no way to know what that meant for V.

He paused. "Paul," he said, "do you think my life has meaning? Did I make the right choices?"

It was stunning: even someone I considered a moral exemplar had these questions in the face of mortality.

V's surgery, chemotherapy, and radiation treatments were trying, but a success. He was back at work a year later, just as I was returning to my clinical duties in the hospital. His hair had thinned and whitened, and the spark in his eyes had dulled. During our final weekly chat, he turned to me and said, "You know, today is the first day it all seems worth it. I mean, obviously, I would've gone through anything for my kids, but today is the first day that all the suffering seems worth it."

How little do doctors understand the hells through which we put patients.

In my sixth year, I returned to the hospital full-time, my research in V's lab now relegated to days off and idle moments, such as they were. Most people, even your closest colleagues, don't quite understand the black hole that is neurosurgical residency. One of my favorite nurses, after sticking around until ten P.M. one night to help us finish a long and difficult case, said to me, "Thank God I have tomorrow off. Do you, too?"

"Um, no."

"But at least you can come in later or something, right? When do you usually get in?"

"Six A.M."

"No. Really?"

"Yep."

"Every day?"

"Every day."

I could see that there were two strategies to cutting the time short, perhaps best exemplified by the tortoise and the hare. The hare moves as fast as possible, hands a blur, instruments clattering, falling to the floor; the skin slips open like a curtain, the skull flap is on the tray before the bone dust settles. As a result, the opening might need to be expanded a centimeter here or there because it's not optimally placed. The tortoise, on the other hand, proceeds deliberately, with no wasted movements, measuring twice, cutting once. No step of the operation needs revisiting; everything moves in a precise, orderly fashion. If the hare makes too many minor missteps and has to keep adjusting, the tortoise wins. If the tortoise spends too much time planning each step, the hare wins.

The funny thing about time in the OR, whether you race frenetically or proceed steadily, is that you have no sense of it passing. If boredom is, as Heidegger argued, the awareness of time passing, then surgery felt like the opposite: the intense focus made the arms of the clock seem arbitrarily placed. Two hours could feel like a minute. Once the final stitch was placed and the wound was dressed, normal time suddenly restarted. You could almost hear an audible *whoosh*. Then you started wondering: How long until the patient wakes up? How long until the next case is rolled in? And what time will I get home tonight?

It wasn't until the last case finished that I felt the length of the day, the drag in my step. Those last few administrative tasks before leaving the hospital were like anvils.

Could it wait until tomorrow?

No.

A sigh, and Earth continued to rotate back toward the sun.

As a chief resident, nearly all responsibility fell on my shoulders, and the opportunities to succeed—or fail— were greater than ever. The pain of failure had led me to understand that technical excellence was a *moral* requirement. Good intentions were not enough, not when so much depended on my skills, when the difference between tragedy and triumph was defined by one or two millimeters.

One day, Matthew, the little boy with the brain tumor who had charmed the ward a few years back, was re-admitted. His hypothalamus had, in fact, been slightly damaged during the operation to remove his tumor; the adorable eight-year-old was now a twelve-year-old monster. He never stopped eating; he threw violent fits. His mother's arms were scarred with purple scratches. Eventually Matthew was institutionalized: he had become a demon, summoned by one millimeter of damage. For every surgery, a family and a surgeon decide together that the benefits outweigh the risks, but this was still heart-breaking. No one wanted to think about what Matthew would be like as a three-hundred-pound twenty-year-old.

Another day, I placed an electrode nine centimeters deep in a patient's brain to treat a Parkinson's tremor. The target was the subthalamic nucleus, a tiny almond-shaped structure deep in the brain. Different parts of it subserve different functions: movement, cognition, emotion. In the operating room, we turned on the current to assess the tremor. With all our eyes on the patient's left hand, we agreed the tremor looked better.

Then the patient's voice, confused, rose above our affirmative murmurs: "I feel . . . overwhelmingly sad."

"Current off!" I said.

"Oh, now the feeling is going away," the patient said.

"Let's recheck the current and impedance, okay? Okay. Current on . . ."

"No, everything . . . it just feels . . . so *sad*. Just dark and, and . . . sad."

"Electrode out!"

We pulled the electrode out and reinserted it, this time two millimeters to the right. The tremor went away. The patient felt, thankfully, fine.

Once, I was doing a late-night case with one of the neurosurgery attendings, a suboccipital craniectomy for a brain-stem malformation. It's one of the most elegant surgeries, in perhaps the most difficult part of the body— just getting there is tricky, no matter how experienced you are. But that night, I felt fluid: the instruments were like extensions of my fingers; the skin, muscle, and bone seemed to unzip themselves; and there I was, staring at a yellow, glistening bulge, a mass deep in the brain stem. Suddenly, the attending stopped me.

"Paul, what happens if you cut two millimeters deeper right here?" He pointed.

Neuroanatomy slides whirred through my head.

"Double vision?"

"No," he said. "Locked-in syndrome." Another two millimeters, and the patient would be completely paralyzed, save for the ability to blink. He didn't look up from the microscope. "And I know this because the third time I did this operation, that's exactly what happened."

Neurosurgery requires a commitment to one's own excellence and a commitment to another's identity. The decision to operate at all involves an appraisal of one's own abilities, as well as a deep sense of who the patient is and what she holds dear. Certain brain areas are considered near-inviolable, like the primary motor cortex, damage to which results in paralysis of affected body parts. But the most sacrosanct regions of the cortex are those that control language. Usually located on the left side, they are called Wernicke's and Broca's areas; one is for understanding language and the other for producing it. Damage to Broca's area results in an inability to speak or write, though the patient can easily understand language. Damage to Wernicke's area results in an inability to understand language; though the patient can still speak, the language she produces is a stream of unconnected words, phrases, and images, a grammar without semantics. If both areas are damaged, the patient becomes an isolate, something central to her humanity stolen forever. After someone suffers a head trauma or a stroke, the destruction of these areas often restrains the surgeon's impulse to save a life: What kind of life exists without language?

When I was a med student, the first patient I met with this sort of problem was a sixty-two-year-old man with a brain tumor. We strolled into his room on morning rounds, and the resident asked him, "Mr. Michaels, how are you feeling today?"

"Four six one eight nineteen!" he replied, somewhat affably.

The tumor had interrupted his speech circuitry, so he could speak only in streams of numbers, but he still had prosody, he could still emote: smile, scowl, sigh. He recited another series of numbers, this time with urgency. There was something he wanted to tell us, but the digits could communicate nothing other than his fear and fury. The team prepared to leave the room; for some reason, I lingered.

"Fourteen one two eight," he pleaded with me, holding my hand. "Fourteen one two eight."

"I'm sorry."

"Fourteen one two eight," he said mournfully, staring into my eyes.

And then I left to catch up to the team. He died a few months later, buried with whatever message he had for the world.

When tumors or malformations abut these language areas, the surgeon takes numerous precautions, ordering a host of different scans, a detailed neuropsychological examination. Critically, however, the surgery is performed with the patient awake and talking. Once the brain is exposed, but before the tumor excision, the surgeon uses a hand-held ball-tip electrode to deliver electrical current to stun a small area of the cortex while the patient performs various verbal tasks: naming objects, reciting the alphabet, and so on. When the electrode sends current into a critical piece of cortex, it disrupts the patient's speech: "A B C D E guh guh guh rrrr . . . F G H I . . ." The brain and the tumor are thus mapped to determine what can be resected safely, and the patient is kept awake throughout, occupied with a combination of formal verbal tasks and small talk.

One evening, as I was prepping for one of these cases,

I reviewed the patient's MRI and noted that the tumor completely covered the language areas. Not a good sign. Reviewing the notes, I saw that the hospital's tumor board—an expert panel of surgeons, oncologists, radiologists, and pathologists—had deemed the case too dangerous for surgery. *How could the surgeon have opted to proceed?* I became a little indignant: at a certain point, it was our job to say no. The patient was wheeled into the room. He fixed his eyes on me and pointed to his head. "I want this *thing* out of my fucking brain. Got it?"

The attending strolled in and saw the expression on my face. "I know," he said. "I tried talking him out of this for about two hours. Don't bother. Ready to go?"

Instead of the usual alphabet recital or counting exercise, we were treated, throughout the surgery, to a litany of profanity and exhortation.

"Is that fucking thing out of my head yet? Why are you slowing down? Go faster! I want it *out.* I can stay here all fucking day, I don't care, just get it out!"

I slowly removed the enormous tumor, attentive to the slightest hint of speech difficulty. With the patient's monologue unceasing, the tumor now sat on a petri dish, his clean brain gleaming.

"Why'd you stop? You some kinda asshole? I told you I want the fucking thing gone!"

"It's done," I said. "It's out."

How was he still talking? Given the size and location of the tumor, it seemed impossible. Profanity supposedly ran on a slightly different circuit from the rest of language. Perhaps the tumor had caused his brain to rewire somehow . . .

But the skull wasn't going to close itself. There would be time for speculation tomorrow.

I had reached the pinnacle of residency. I had mastered the core operations. My research had garnered the highest awards. Job interest was trickling in from all over the country. Stanford launched a search for a position that fit my interests exactly, for a neurosurgeon-neuroscientist focused on techniques of neural modulation. One of my junior residents came up to me and said, "I just heard from the bosses—if they hire you, you're going to be my faculty mentor!"

"Shhhh," I said. "Don't jinx it."

It felt to me as if the individual strands of biology,

morality, life, and death were finally beginning to weave themselves into, if not a perfect moral system, a coherent worldview and a sense of my place in it. Doctors in highly charged fields met patients at inflected moments, the most authentic moments, where life and identity were under threat; their duty included learning what made that particular patient's life worth living, and planning to save those things if possible—or to allow the peace of death if not. Such power required deep responsibility, sharing in guilt and recrimination.

I was at a conference in San Diego when my phone rang. My co-resident, Victoria.

"Paul?"

Something was wrong. My stomach tightened.

"What's up?" I said.

Silence.

"Vic?"

"It's Jeff. He killed himself."

"*What?*"

Jeff was finishing his surgical fellowship in the Midwest, and we were both so punishingly busy . . . we'd lost touch. I tried to recall our last conversation and couldn't.

"He, uh—he apparently had a difficult complication,

and his patient died. Last night he climbed onto the roof of a building and jumped off. I don't really know anything else."

I searched for a question to bring understanding. None was forthcoming. I could only imagine the overwhelming guilt, like a tidal wave, that had lifted him up and off that building.

I wished, desperately, that I could've been walking with him out the door of the hospital that evening. I wished we could've commiserated as we used to. I wished I could have told Jeff what I had come to understand about life, and our chosen way of life, if only to hear his wise, clever counsel. Death comes for all of us. For us, for our patients: it is our fate as living, breathing, metabolizing organisms. Most lives are lived with passivity toward death—it's something that happens to you and those around you. But Jeff and I had trained for years to actively engage with death, to grapple with it, like Jacob with the angel, and, in so doing, to confront the meaning of a life. We had assumed an onerous yoke, that of *mortal responsibility*. Our patients' lives and identities may be in our hands, yet death always wins. Even if you are perfect, the world isn't. The secret is to know that the deck is stacked, that you will lose, that your hands or judgment will slip, and yet still struggle to win for your patients. You can't ever reach perfection, but you can believe in an asymptote toward which you are ceaselessly striving.

PART II

Cease Not till Death

LYING NEXT TO LUCY in the hospital bed, both of us crying, the CT scan images still glowing on the computer screen, that identity as a physician—my identity—no longer mattered. With the cancer having invaded multiple organ systems, the diagnosis was clear. The room was quiet. Lucy told me she loved me. "I don't want to die," I said. I told her to remarry, that I couldn't bear the thought of her being alone. I told her we should refinance the mortgage immediately. We started calling family members. At some point, Victoria came by the room, and we discussed the scan and the likely future treatments. When she brought up the logistics of returning to residency, I stopped her.

"Victoria," I said, "I'm never coming back to this hospital as a doctor. Don't you think?"

One chapter of my life seemed to have ended; perhaps the whole book was closing. Instead of being the pastoral figure aiding a life transition, I found myself the sheep, lost and confused. Severe illness wasn't life-altering, it was life-shattering. It felt less like an epiphany—a piercing burst of light, illuminating What Really Matters—and more like someone had just firebombed the path forward. Now I would have to work around it.

My brother Jeevan had arrived at my bedside. "You've accomplished so much," he said. "You know that, don't you?"

I sighed. He meant well, but the words rang hollow. My life had been building potential, potential that would now go unrealized. I had planned to do so much, and I had come so close. I was physically debilitated, my imagined future and my personal identity collapsed, and I faced the same existential quandaries my patients faced. The lung cancer diagnosis was confirmed. My carefully planned and hard-won future no longer existed. Death, so familiar to me in my work, was now paying a personal visit. Here we were, finally face-to-face, and yet nothing about it seemed recognizable. Standing at the crossroads where I should have been able to see and follow the footprints of the countless patients I had treated over the years, I saw instead only a blank, a harsh, vacant, gleaming white desert, as if a sandstorm had erased all trace of familiarity.

The sun was setting. I would be discharged the next morning. An oncology appointment was set for later in the week, but the nurse told me my oncologist was going to drop by that night, before leaving to pick up her kids. Her name was Emma Hayward, and she wanted to say hello before the initial office visit. I knew Emma a little— I had treated some of her patients before—but we had never spoken beyond passing professional courtesies. My parents and brothers were scattered about the room, not saying much, while Lucy sat by the bed, holding my hand. The door opened and in she walked, her white coat showing the wear of a long day but her smile fresh. Trailing behind her were her fellow and a resident. Emma was only a few years older than I, her hair long and dark, but as is common to all those who spend time with death, streaked with gray. She pulled up a chair.

"Hi, my name is Emma," she said. "I'm sorry to have to be so brief today, but I wanted to come by and introduce myself."

We shook hands, my arm entangled in the IV line.

"Thanks for stopping by," I said. "I know you have kids to pick up. This is my family." She nodded hello at Lucy, at my brothers and parents.

"I'm sorry this is happening to you," she said. "To all of you. There will be a lot of time to talk in a couple days. I went ahead and had the lab start running some tests on your tumor sample, which will help guide therapy. Treatment may be chemotherapy or not, depending on the tests."

Eighteen months earlier, I'd been in the hospital with appendicitis. Then I'd been treated not as a patient but as a colleague, almost like a consultant on my own case. I expected the same here. "I know now's not the time," I proceeded, "but I will want to talk about the Kaplan-Meier survival curves."

"No," she said. "Absolutely not."

A brief silence. *How dare she?* I thought. *This is how doctors—doctors like me—understand prognostication. I have a right to know.*

"We can talk about therapies later," she said. "We can talk about your going back to work, too, if that's what you'd like to do. The traditional chemotherapy combination—cisplatin, pemetrexed, possibly with Avastin, too—has a high rate of peripheral neuropathy, so we'd probably switch the cisplatin for carboplatin, which will protect your nerves better, since you're a surgeon."

Go back to work? What is she talking about? Is she delusional? Or am I dead wrong about my prognosis? And how can we talk about any of this without a realistic estimate of survival? The ground, having already buckled and roiled over the past few days, did so again.

"We can do details later," she continued, "as I know this is a lot to absorb. Mostly, I just wanted to meet you all before our appointment Thursday. Is there anything I can do, or answer—besides survival curves—today?"

"No," I said, my mind reeling. "Thanks so much for stopping by. I really appreciate it."

"Here's my card," she said, "and there's the clinic number. Feel free to call if anything comes up before we see you in two days."

My family and friends quickly wired through our network of medical colleagues to find out who the best lung cancer oncologists in the country were. Houston and New York had major cancer centers; was that where I should be treated? The logistics of moving or temporarily relocating or what have you—that could be sorted out later. The replies came back quickly, and more or less unanimously: Emma not only was one of the best— a world-renowned oncologist who served as the lung cancer expert on one of the major national cancer advisory boards—but she was also known to be compassionate, someone who knew when to push and when to hold back. I briefly wondered at the string of events that had sent me looping through the world, my residency determined by a computerized match process, only to end up assigned here, with a freak diagnosis, in the hands of one of the finest doctors to treat it.

Having spent the better part of the week bedridden, with the cancer progressing, I had grown noticeably weaker. My body, and the identity tied to it, had radically changed. No longer was getting in and out of bed to go to the bathroom an automated subcortical motor program; it took effort and planning. The physical therapists left a list of items to ease my transition home: a cane, a modified toilet seat, foam blocks for leg support while resting. A bevy of new pain medications was prescribed. As I hobbled out of the hospital, I wondered how, just six days ago, I had spent nearly thirty-six straight hours in the operating room. Had I grown that much sicker in a week? Yes, in part. But I had also used a number of tricks and help from co-surgeons to get through those thirty-six hours—and, even so, I had suffered excruciating pain. Had the confirmation of my fears—in the CT scan, in the lab results, both showing not merely cancer but a body overwhelmed, nearing death—released me from the duty to serve, from my duty to patients, to neurosurgery, to the pursuit of goodness? Yes, I thought, and therein was the paradox: like a runner crossing the finish line only to collapse, without that duty to care for the ill pushing me forward, I became an invalid.

Usually when I had a patient with a strange condition, I consulted the relevant specialist and spent time reading about it. This seemed no different, but as I started reading about chemo, which included a whole variety of agents, and a raft of more modern novel treatments that targeted specific mutations, the sheer number of questions I had prevented any useful directed study. (Alexander Pope: "A little learning is a dangerous thing; / Drink deep, or taste not the Pierian spring.") Without appropriate medical experience, I couldn't place myself in this new world of information, couldn't find my spot on the Kaplan-Meier curve. I waited, expectantly, for my clinic visit.

But mostly, I rested.

I sat, staring at a photo of Lucy and me from medical school, dancing and laughing; it was so sad, those two, planning a life together, unaware, never suspecting their own fragility. My friend Laurie had had a fiancé when she'd died in a car accident—was this any crueler?

My family engaged in a flurry of activity to transform my life from that of a doctor to that of a patient. We set up an account with a mail-order pharmacy, ordered a bed rail, and bought an ergonomic mattress to help alleviate the searing back pain. Our financial plan, which a few days before had banked on my income increasing sixfold in the next year, now looked precarious, and a variety of new financial instruments seemed necessary to protect Lucy. My father declared that these modifications were capitulations to the disease: I was going to beat this thing, I would somehow be cured. How often had I heard a patient's family member make similar declarations? I never knew what to say to them then, and I didn't know what to say to my father now.

What was the alternate story?

Two days later, Lucy and I met Emma in the clinic. My parents hovered in the waiting room. The medical assistant took my vitals. Emma and her nurse practitioner were remarkably punctual, and Emma pulled up a chair in front of me, to talk face-to-face, eye-to-eye.

"Hello again," she said. "This is Alexis, my right hand." She gestured to the NP, who sat at the computer taking notes. "I know there's a lot to discuss, but first: How are you doing?"

"Okay, all things considered," I said. "Enjoying my 'vacation,' I guess. How are you?"

"Oh, I'm okay." She paused—patients don't typically

ask how their doctors are doing, but Emma was also a colleague. "I'm running the inpatient service this week, so you know how that is." She smiled. Lucy and I *did* know. Outpatient specialists rotated on the inpatient service periodically, adding several hours of work in an already jam-packed day.

After more pleasantries, we settled into a comfortable discussion on the state of lung cancer research. There were two paths forward, she said. The traditional method was chemotherapy, which generically targeted rapidly dividing cells—primarily cancer cells but also cells in your bone marrow, hair follicles, intestines, and so forth. Emma reviewed the data and options, lecturing as if to another doctor—but again with the exception of any mention of Kaplan-Meier survival curves. Newer therapies had been developed, however, targeting specific molecular defects in the cancer itself. I had heard rumors of such efforts—it had long been a holy grail in cancer work—and was surprised to learn how much progress had been made. These treatments, it seemed, had led to long-term survival in "some" patients.

"Most of your tests are back," Emma said. "You have a PI3K mutation, but no one's sure what that means yet.

The test for the most common mutation in patients like you, EGFR, is still pending. I'm betting that's what you have, and if so, there's a pill called Tarceva that you can take instead of chemotherapy. That result should be back tomorrow, Friday, but you're sick enough that I've set you up for chemo starting Monday in case the EGFR test is negative."

I immediately felt a kinship. This was exactly how I approached neurosurgery: have a plan A, B, and C at all times.

"With chemo, our main decision will be carboplatin versus cisplatin. In isolated studies, head-to-head, carboplatin is better tolerated. Cisplatin has potentially better results but much worse toxicity, especially for the nerves, though all the data is old, and there's no direct comparison within our modern chemo regimens. Do you have any thoughts?"

"I'm less worried about protecting my hands for surgery," I said. "There's a lot I can do with my life. If I lose my hands, I can find another job, or not work, or something."

She paused. "Let me ask this: Is surgery *important* to you? Is it something you want to do?"

"Well, yes, I've spent almost a third of my life preparing for it."

"Okay, then I'm going to suggest we stick with the carboplatin. I don't think it will change survival, and I do think it could dramatically change your quality of life. Do you have any other questions?"

She seemed clear that this was the way to go, and I was happy to follow. Maybe, I began to let myself believe, performing surgery again was a possibility. I felt myself relax a little.

"Can I start smoking?" I joked.

Lucy laughed, and Emma rolled her eyes.

"No. Any *serious* questions?"

"The Kaplan-Meier—"

"We're not discussing that," she said.

I didn't understand her resistance. After all, I was a doctor familiar with these statistics. I could look them up myself . . . so that's what I would have to do.

"Okay," I said, "then I think everything is pretty clear. We'll hear from you tomorrow about the EGFR results. If yes, then we'll start a pill, Tarceva. If no, then we start chemotherapy Monday."

"Right. The other thing I want you to know is this: I

am your doctor now. Any problem you have, from primary care to whatever, you come to us first."

Again, I felt a pang of kinship.

"Thanks," I said. "And good luck on the inpatient wards."

She left the room, only to pop her head back in a second later. "Feel free to say no to this, but there are some lung cancer fundraisers who would love to meet you. Don't answer now—think about it, and let Alexis know if you might be interested. Don't do anything you don't want to."

As we left, Lucy remarked, "She's great. She's a good fit for you. Although . . ." She smiled. "I think she likes you."

"And?"

"Well, there's that study that says doctors do a worse job prognosticating for patients they're personally invested in."

"On our list of things to worry about," I said, with a laugh, "I think that's in the bottom quartile."

I began to realize that coming in such close contact with my own mortality had changed both nothing and everything. Before my cancer was diagnosed, I knew that someday I would die, but I didn't know when. After the diagnosis, I knew that someday I would die, but I didn't know when. But now I knew it acutely. The problem wasn't really a scientific one. The fact of death is unsettling. Yet there is no other way to live.

Slowly the medical fog was clearing—at least now I had enough information to dive into the literature. While the numbers were fuzzy, having an EGFR mutation seemed to add around a year of life on average, with the potential for long-term survival; not having it suggested an 80 percent chance of death within two years. Clarifying the rest of my life was going to be a process.

The next day, Lucy and I went to the sperm bank, to preserve gametes and options. We had always planned to have kids at the end of my residency, but now . . . The cancer drugs would have an unknown effect on my sperm, so to keep a chance of having children, we'd have to freeze sperm before I started treatment. A young woman walked us through a variety of payment plans and options for storage and legal forms for ownership. On her desk were a multitude of colorful pamphlets about various social outings for young people with cancer: improv groups, a cappella groups, open-mike nights, and so on. I envied their happy faces, knowing that, statistically, they all probably had highly treatable forms of cancer, and reasonable life expectancies. Only 0.0012 percent of thirty-six-year-olds get lung cancer. Yes, all cancer patients are unlucky, but there's cancer, and then there's *CANCER*, and you have to be really unlucky to have the latter. When she asked us to specify what would happen to the sperm if one of us "were to die"—who would legally own them in the event of death—tears began rolling down Lucy's face.

The word *hope* first appeared in English about a thousand years ago, denoting some combination of confidence and desire. But what I desired—life—was not what I was confident about—death. When I talked about hope, then, did I really mean "Leave some room for unfounded desire?" No. Medical statistics not only describe numbers such as mean survival, they measure our confidence in our numbers, with tools like confidence levels, confidence intervals, and confidence bounds. So did I mean "Leave some room for a statistically improbable but still plausible outcome—a survival just above the measured 95 percent confidence interval?" Is that what hope was? Could we divide the curve into existential sections, from "defeated" to "pessimistic" to "realistic" to "hopeful" to "delusional"? Weren't the numbers just the numbers? Had we all just given in to the "hope" that every patient was above average?

It occurred to me that my relationship with statistics changed as soon as I became one.

During my residency, I had sat with countless patients and families to discuss grim prognoses; it's one of the most important jobs you have, as a physician. It's easier when the patient is ninety-four, in the last stages of dementia, with a severe brain bleed. But for someone like me—a thirty-six-year-old given a diagnosis of terminal cancer—there aren't really words.

The reason doctors don't give patients specific prognoses is not merely because they cannot. Certainly, if a patient's expectations are way out of the bounds of probability—someone expecting to live to 130, say, or someone thinking his benign skin spots are signs of imminent death—doctors are entrusted to bring that person's expectations into the realm of reasonable possibility. What patients seek is not scientific knowledge that doctors hide but existential authenticity each person must find on her own. Getting too deeply into statistics is like trying to quench a thirst with salty water. The angst of facing mortality has no remedy in probability.

When we arrived home from the sperm bank, I got a phone call saying that I did, in fact, have a treatable mutation (EGFR). Chemo was off, thankfully, and Tarceva, a little white pill, became my treatment. I soon began to feel stronger. And even though I no longer really knew what it was, I felt it: a drop of hope. The fog surrounding my life rolled back another inch, and a sliver of blue sky peeked through. In the weeks that followed, my appetite returned. I put on a little weight. I developed the characteristic severe acne that correlates with a good response. Lucy had always loved my smooth skin, but now it was pockmarked and, with my blood thinners, constantly bleeding. Any part of me that identified with being handsome was slowly being erased—though, in fairness, I was happy to be uglier and alive. Lucy said she loved my skin just the same, acne and all, but while I knew that our identities derive not just from the brain, I was living its embodied nature. The man who loved hiking, camping, and running, who expressed his love through gigantic hugs, who threw his giggling niece high in the air—that was a man I no longer was. At best, I could aim to be him again.

At our first of several biweekly appointments, Emma's and my discussion tended from the medical ("How's the rash?") to the more existential. The traditional cancer narrative—that one ought to recede, spend time with family, and settle one's toes in the peat—was one option.

"Many people, once diagnosed, quit work entirely," she said. "Others focus on it heavily. Either way is okay."

"I had mapped out this whole forty-year career for myself—the first twenty as a surgeon-scientist, the last twenty as a writer. But now that I am likely well into my last twenty years, I don't know which career I should be pursuing."

"Well, I can't tell you that," she said. "I can only say that you *can* get back to surgery if you want, but you have to figure out what's most important to you."

"If I had some sense of how much time I have left, it'd

be easier. If I had two years, I'd write. If I had ten, I'd get back to surgery and science."

"You know I can't give you a number."

Yes, I knew. It was up to me, to quote her oft-repeated refrain, to find my values. Part of me felt this was a cop-out: okay, fine, I never gave out specific numbers to patients, either, but didn't I always have a sense of how the patient would do? How else did I make life-and-death decisions? Then I recalled the times I had been wrong: the time I had counseled a family to withdraw life support for their son, only for the parents to appear two years later, showing me a YouTube video of him playing piano, and delivering cupcakes in thanks for saving his life.

My oncology appointments were the most important of many new appointments with a variety of healthcare providers, but they weren't the only ones. At Lucy's insistence, we began seeing a couples therapist who specialized in cancer patients. Sitting in her windowless office, in side-by-side armchairs, Lucy and I detailed the ways in which our lives, present and future, had been fractured by my diagnosis, and the pain of knowing and not knowing the future, the difficulty in planning, the necessity of being there for each other. In truth, cancer had helped save our marriage.

"Well, you two are coping with this better than any couple I've seen," the therapist said at the end of our first session. "I'm not sure I have any advice for you."

I laughed as we walked out—at least I was excelling at something again. The years of ministering to terminally ill patients had borne some fruit! I turned to Lucy, expecting to see a smile; instead, she was shaking her head.

"Don't you get it?" she said, taking my hand in hers. "If we're the best at this, *that means it doesn't get better than this.*"

If the weight of mortality does not grow lighter, does it at least get more familiar?

Once I had been diagnosed with a terminal illness, I began to view the world through two perspectives; I was starting to see death as both doctor and patient. As a doctor, I knew not to declare "Cancer is a battle I'm going to win!" or ask "Why me?" (Answer: Why *not* me?) I knew a lot about medical care, complications, and treatment algorithms. I quickly learned from my oncologist

The bulk of my week was spent not in cognitive therapy but in physical therapy. I had sent nearly every one of my patients to physical therapy. And now I found myself shocked at how difficult it was. As a doctor, you have a sense of what it's like to be sick, but until you've gone through it yourself, you don't really know. It's like falling in love or having a kid. You don't appreciate the mounds of paperwork that come along with it, or the little things. When you get an IV placed, for example, you can actually taste the salt when they start infusing it. They tell me that this happens to everybody, but even after eleven years in medicine, I had never known.

In physical therapy, I was not even lifting weights yet, just lifting my legs. This was exhausting and humiliating. My brain was fine, but I did not feel like myself. My body was frail and weak—the person who could run half marathons was a distant memory—and that, too, shapes your identity. Racking back pain can mold an identity; fatigue and nausea can, as well. Karen, my PT, asked me what my goals were. I picked two: riding my bike and going for a run. In the face of weakness, determination set in. Day after day I kept at it, and every tiny increase in strength broadened the possible worlds, the possible versions of me. I started adding reps, weights, and minutes to my workouts, pushing myself to the point of vomiting. After two months, I could sit for thirty minutes without tiring. I could start going to dinner with friends again.

One afternoon, Lucy and I drove down to Cañada Road, our favorite biking spot. (Usually we would bike there, pride forces me to add, but the hills were still too formidable for my lightweight frame.) I managed six wobbly miles. It was a far cry from the breezy, thirty-mile rides of the previous summer, but at least I could balance on two wheels.

Was this a victory or a defeat?

I began to look forward to my meetings with Emma. In her office, I felt like myself, like *a* self. Outside her office, I no longer knew who I was. Because I wasn't working, I didn't feel like myself, a neurosurgeon, a scientist— a young man, relatively speaking, with a bright future spread before him. Debilitated, at home, I feared I wasn't much of a husband for Lucy. I had passed from the subject to the direct object of every sentence of my life. In fourteenth-century philosophy, the word *patient* simply meant "the object of an action," and I felt like one. As a doctor, I was an agent, a cause; as a patient, I was merely something to which things happened. But in Emma's office, Lucy and I could joke, trade doctor lingo, talk freely about our hopes and dreams, try to assemble a plan to move forward. Two months in, Emma remained vague about any prognostication, and every statistic I cited she rebuffed with a reminder to focus on my values. Though I felt dissatisfied, at least I felt like somebody, a person, rather than a thing exemplifying the second law of thermodynamics (all order tends toward entropy, decay, etc.).

Flush in the face of mortality, many decisions became compressed, urgent and unreceding. Foremost among them for us: Should Lucy and I have a child? Even if our marriage had been strained toward the end of my residency, we had always remained very much in love. Our relationship was still deep in meaning, a shared and evolving vocabulary about what mattered. If human relationality formed the bedrock of meaning, it seemed to us that rearing children added another dimension to that meaning. It had been something we'd always wanted, and we were both impelled by the instinct to do it still, to add another chair to our family's table.

Both of us yearning to be parents, we each thought of

the other. Lucy hoped I had years left, but understanding my prognosis, she felt that the choice—whether to spend my remaining time as a father—should be mine.

"What are you most afraid or sad about?" she asked me one night as we were lying in bed.

"Leaving you," I told her.

I knew a child would bring joy to the whole family, and I couldn't bear to picture Lucy husbandless and childless after I died, but I was adamant that the decision ultimately be hers: she would likely have to raise the child on her own, after all, and to care for both of us as my illness progressed.

"Will having a newborn distract from the time we have together?" she asked. "Don't you think saying goodbye to your child will make your death *more* painful?"

"Wouldn't it be great if it did?" I said. Lucy and I both felt that life wasn't about avoiding suffering.

Years ago, it had occurred to me that Darwin and Nietzsche agreed on one thing: the defining characteristic of the organism is striving. Describing life otherwise was like painting a tiger without stripes. After so many years of living with death, I'd come to understand that the easiest death wasn't necessarily the best. We talked it over. Our families gave their blessing. We decided to have a child. We would carry on living, instead of dying.

Because of the medications I was on, assisted reproduction appeared to be the only route forward. So we visited a specialist at a reproductive endocrinology clinic in Palo Alto. She was efficient and professional, but her lack of experience dealing with terminally ill, as opposed to infertile, patients was obvious. She plowed through her spiel, eyes on her clipboard:

"How long have you been trying?"

"Well, we haven't yet."

"Oh, right. Of course."

Finally she asked, "Given your, uh, *situation,* I assume you want to get pregnant fast?"

"Yes," Lucy said. "We'd like to start right away."

"I'd suggest you begin with IVF, then," she said.

When I mentioned that we'd rather minimize how many embryos were created and destroyed, she looked slightly confused. Most people who came here prized expedience above all. But I was determined to avoid the situation where, after I died, Lucy had responsibility for a half dozen embryos—the last remnants of our shared genomes, my last presence on this earth—stuck in a freezer somewhere, too painful to destroy, impossible to bring to full humanity: technological artifacts that no one knew how to relate to. But after several trials of intrauterine insemination, it was clear we needed a higher level of technology: we would need to create at least a few embryos in vitro and implant the healthiest. The others would die. Even in having children in this new life, death played its part.

Six weeks after starting treatment, I was due for my first CT scan to measure the efficacy of the Tarceva. As I hopped out of the scanner, the CT tech looked at me. "Well, Doc," he offered, "I'm not supposed to say this, but there's a computer back there if you want to take a look." I loaded up the images on the viewer, typing in my own name.

The acne was a reassuring sign. My strength had also improved, though I was still limited by back pain and fatigue. Sitting there, I reminded myself of what Emma had said: even a small amount of tumor growth, so long as it was small, would be considered a success.

(My father, of course, had predicted that all the cancer would be gone. "Your scan will be clear, Pubby!" he'd declared, using my family nickname.) I repeated to myself that even small growth was good news, took a breath, and clicked. The images materialized on the screen. My lungs, speckled with innumerable tumors before, were clear except for a one-centimeter nodule in the right upper lobe. I could make out my spine beginning to heal. There had been a clear, dramatic reduction in tumor burden.

Relief washed over me.

My cancer was stable.

When we met Emma the next day she still refused to talk prognosis, but she said, "You're well enough that we can meet every six weeks now. Next time we meet, we can start to talk about what your life might be like." I could feel the chaos of the past months receding, a sense of a new order settling in. My contracted sense of the future began to relax.

A local meeting of former Stanford neurosurgery graduates was happening that weekend, and I looked forward to the chance to reconnect with my former self. Yet being there merely heightened the surreal contrast of what my life was now. I was surrounded by success and possibility and ambition, by peers and seniors whose lives were running along a trajectory that was no longer mine, whose bodies could still tolerate standing for a grueling eight-hour surgery. I felt trapped inside a reversed Christmas carol: Victoria was opening the happy present—grants, job offers, publications—I should be sharing. My senior peers were living the future that was no longer mine: early career awards, promotions, new houses.

No one asked about my plans, which was a relief, since I had none. While I could now walk without a cane, a paralytic uncertainty loomed: Who would I be, going forward, and for how long? Invalid, scientist, teacher? Bioethicist? Neurosurgeon once again, as Emma had implied? Stay-at-home dad? Writer? Who could, or should, I be? As a doctor, I had had some sense of what patients with life-changing illnesses faced—and it was exactly these moments I had wanted to explore with them. Shouldn't terminal illness, then, be the perfect gift to that young man who had wanted to understand death? What better way to understand it than to live it? But I'd had no idea how hard it would be, how much terrain I would have to explore, map, settle. I'd always imagined the doctor's work as something like connecting two pieces of railroad track, allowing a smooth journey for the patient. I hadn't expected the prospect of facing my own mortality to be so disorienting, so dislocating. I thought back to my younger self, who might've wanted to "forge in the smithy of my soul the uncreated conscience of my race"; looking into my own soul, I found the tools too brittle, the fire too weak, to forge even my own conscience.

Lost in a featureless wasteland of my own mortality, and finding no traction in the reams of scientific studies, intracellular molecular pathways, and endless curves of survival statistics, I began reading literature again: Solzhenitsyn's *Cancer Ward*, B. S. Johnson's *The Unfortunates*, Tolstoy's *Ivan Ilyich*, Nagel's *Mind and Cosmos*, Woolf, Kafka, Montaigne, Frost, Greville, memoirs of cancer patients—anything by anyone who had ever written about mortality. I was searching for a vocabulary with which to make sense of death, to find a way to begin defining myself and inching forward again. The privilege of direct experience had led me away from literary and academic work, yet now I felt that to understand my own direct experiences, I would have to translate them back into language. Hemingway described his process in similar terms: acquiring rich experiences, then retreating to cogitate and write about them. I needed words to go forward.

And so it was literature that brought me back to life during this time. The monolithic uncertainty of my future was deadening; everywhere I turned, the shadow of death obscured the meaning of any action. I remember the moment when my overwhelming unease yielded, when that seemingly impassable sea of uncertainty parted. I woke up in pain, facing another day—no project beyond breakfast seemed tenable. *I can't go on,* I thought, and immediately, its antiphon responded, completing Samuel Beckett's seven words, words I had learned long ago as an undergraduate: *I'll go on.* I got out of bed and took a step forward, repeating the phrase over and over: "I can't go on. I'll go on."

That morning, I made a decision: I would push myself to return to the OR. Why? Because I could. Because that's who I was. Because I would have to learn to live in a different way, seeing death as an imposing itinerant visitor but knowing that even if I'm dying, until I actually die, I am still living.

Over the next six weeks, I altered my physical therapy program, focusing now on building strength specifically for operating: long hours of standing, micromanipulation of small objects, pronation for placing pedicle screws.

Another CT scan followed. The tumor had shrunk slightly more. Going over the images with me, Emma said, "I don't know how long you've got, but I will say this: the patient I saw just before you today has been on Tarceva for seven years without a problem. You've still got a ways to go before we're that comfortable with your cancer. But, looking at you, thinking about living ten years is not crazy. You might not make it, but it's not crazy."

Here was the prognostication—no, not prognostication: justification. Justification of my decision to return to neurosurgery, to return to life. One part of me exulted at the prospect of ten years. Another part wished she'd said, "Going back to being a neurosurgeon is crazy for you—pick something easier." I was startled to realize that in spite of everything, the last few months had had one area of lightness: not having to bear the tremendous weight of the responsibility neurosurgery demanded—and part of me wanted to be excused from picking up the yoke again. Neurosurgery is really hard work, and no one would have faulted me for not going back. (People often ask if it is a calling, and my answer is always yes. You can't see it as a job, because if it's a job, it's one of the worst jobs there is.) A couple of my professors actively discouraged the idea: "Shouldn't you be spending time with your family?" ("Shouldn't *you*?" I wondered. I was making the decision to do this work because this work, to me, was a sacred thing.) Lucy and I had just reached the top of the hill, the landmarks of Silicon Valley, buildings bearing the names of every biomedical and technological transformation of the last generation, unfolding below us. Eventually, though, the itch to hold a surgical drill again had become too compelling. Moral duty has weight, things that have weight have gravity, and so the duty to bear mortal responsibility pulled me back into the operating room. Lucy was fully supportive.

I called up the program director to tell him I was ready to return. He was thrilled. Victoria and I talked about how best to reintroduce me and get me back up to speed. I requested that a fellow resident be available to back me up at all times in case something went awry. Furthermore, I would do only one case per day. I wouldn't manage the patients outside the OR or be on call. We'd proceed conservatively. The OR schedule came out, and I was assigned to a temporal lobectomy, one of my favorite operations. Commonly, epilepsy is caused by a misfiring hippocampus, which is located deep in the temporal lobe. Removing the hippocampus can cure the epilepsy, but the operation is complex, requiring gentle dissection of the hippocampus off the pia, the delicate transparent covering of the brain, right near the brain stem.

I spent the night prior poring through surgical textbooks, reviewing the anatomy and steps of the operation. I slept restlessly, seeing the angle of the head, the saw against the skull, the way the light reflects off the pia once the temporal lobe is removed. I got out of bed and put on a shirt and tie. (I had returned all my scrubs months ago, assuming I'd never need them again.) I arrived at the hospital and changed into the familiar blue garb for the first time in eighteen weeks. I chatted with the patient to make sure there were no last-minute questions, then began the process of setting up the OR. The patient was intubated, the attending and I were scrubbed and ready to begin. I picked up the scalpel and incised the skin just above the ear, proceeding slowly, trying to make sure I forgot nothing and made no mistakes. With the electrocautery, I deepened the incision to the bone, then elevated the skin flap with hooks. Everything felt familiar, muscle memory kicking in. I took the drill and made three holes in the skull. The attending squirted water to keep the drill cool as I worked. Switching to the craniotome, a sideways-cutting drill bit, I connected the holes, freeing up a large piece of bone. With a crack, I pried it off. There lay the silvery dura. Happily, I hadn't damaged it with the drill, a common beginner's mistake. I used a sharp knife to open the dura without injuring the brain. Success again. I began to relax. I tacked back the dura with small stitches to keep it out of the way of the main surgery. The brain gently pulsed and glis-

little more slowly. On day three, I was removing a degenerated disc from a patient's spine. I stared at the bulging disc, not remembering my exact move. The fellow supervising me suggested taking small bites with a rongeur.

"Yeah, I know that's how it's usually done," I mumbled, "but there's another way . . ."

I nibbled away for twenty minutes, my brain searching for the more elegant way I had learned to do this. At the next spinal level, it came back to me in a flash.

"Cobb instrument!" I called out. "Mallet. Kerrison."

I had the whole disc removed in thirty seconds. "That's how I do this," I said.

Over the next couple of weeks, my strength continued to improve, as did my fluency and technique. My hands relearned how to manipulate submillimeter blood vessels without injury, my fingers conjuring up the old tricks they'd once known. After a month, I was operating a nearly full load.

I kept myself limited to operating, leaving the administration, patient care, and night and weekend calls to Victoria and the other senior residents. I had already mastered those skills, anyway, and needed to learn only the nuances of complex operations to feel complete. I ended my days exhausted beyond measure, muscles on fire, slowly improving. But the truth was, it was joyless. The visceral pleasure I'd once found in operating was gone, replaced by an iron focus on overcoming the nausea, the pain, the fatigue. Coming home each night, I would scarf down a handful of pain pills, then crawl into bed next to Lucy, who had returned to a full work schedule as well. She was now in the first trimester of pregnancy, with the baby due in June, when I would complete residency. We had a photo of our child as a blastocyst, taken just before implantation. ("She has your cell membrane," I remarked to Lucy.) Still, I was determined to restore my life to its prior trajectory.

Another stable scan six months after diagnosis passed, and I reopened my job search. With my cancer under control, I might have several years left. It seemed the career I had worked for years to attain, which had disappeared amid disease, was now back in reach. I could almost hear trumpets sounding a victory fanfare.

· · ·

During my next visit with Emma, we talked about life and where it was taking me. I recalled Henry Adams trying to compare the scientific force of the combustion engine and the existential force of the Virgin Mary. The scientific questions were settled for now, allowing the existential ones full play, yet both were in the doctor's purview. I had recently learned that the surgeon-scientist position at Stanford—the job for which I had been heir apparent—had been filled while I was out sick. I was crushed, and told her so.

"Well," she said, "this doctor-professor thing can be a real grind. But you know that already. I'm sorry."

"Yeah, I guess the science that excited me was about twenty-year projects. Without that kind of time frame, I'm not sure I'm all that interested in being a scientist." I tried to console myself. "You can't get much done in a couple of years."

"Right. And just remember, you're doing great. You're working again. You've got a baby on the way. You're finding your values, and that's not easy."

Later that day one of the younger professors, a former resident and close friend, stopped me in the hallway.

"Hey," she said. "There's been a lot of discussion in faculty meetings about what to do with you."

"What to do with me, how?"

"I think some professors are concerned about you graduating."

Graduation from residency required two things: meeting a set of national and local requirements, which I'd already done, and the blessing of the faculty.

"What?" I said. "I don't mean to sound cocky, but I'm a good surgeon, just as good as—"

"I know. I think they probably just want to see you performing the full load of a chief. It's because they like you. Seriously."

I realized it was true: For the past few months, I had been acting merely as a surgical technician. I had been using cancer as an excuse not to take full responsibility for my patients. On the other hand, it was a good excuse, damn it. But now I started coming in earlier, staying later, fully caring for the patients again, adding another four hours to a twelve-hour day. It put the patients back in the center of my mind at all times. The first two days I thought I would have to quit, battling waves of nausea, pain, and fatigue, retreating to an unused bed in down moments to sleep. But by the third day, I had begun to enjoy it again, despite the wreck of my body. Reconnecting with patients brought back the meaning of this work. I took antiemetics and nonsteroidal anti-inflammatory drugs (NSAIDs) between cases and just before rounds. I was suffering, but I was fully back. Instead of finding an unused bed, I started resting on the junior residents' couch, supervising them on the care of my patients, lecturing as I rode a wave of back spasms. The more tortured my body became, the more I relished having done the work. At the end of the first week, I slept for forty hours straight.

But I was calling the shots:

"Hey, boss," I said, "I was just reviewing cases for tomorrow, and I know the first case is booked interhemispheric, but I think it will be much safer and easier if we come parietal transcortical."

"Really?" the attending said. "Let me look at the films. . . . You know what? You're right. Can you change the booking?"

The next day: "Hi, sir, it's Paul. I just saw Mr. F and his family in the ICU—I think we'll need to take him tomorrow for an ACDF. Okay if I book it? When are you free?"

And I was back to full speed in the OR:

"Nurse, can you page Dr. S? I'm going to be done with this case before he gets here."

"I've got him on the phone. He says you can't possibly be done yet."

The attending came running in, out of breath, scrubbed, and peered through the microscope.

"I took a slightly acute angle to avoid the sinus," I said, "but the whole tumor's out."

"You avoided the sinus?"

"Yes, sir."

"You got it out in one piece?"

"Yes, sir, it's on the table so you can have a look."

"Looks good. Really good. When did you get to be so fast? Sorry I wasn't here earlier."

"No trouble."

The tricky part of illness is that, as you go through it, your values are constantly changing. You try to figure out what matters to you, and then you keep figuring it out. It felt like someone had taken away my credit card and I was having to learn how to budget. You may decide you want to spend your time working as a neurosurgeon, but two months later, you may feel differently. Two months after that, you may want to learn to play the saxophone or devote yourself to the church. Death may be a one-time event, but living with terminal illness is a process.

It struck me that I had traversed the five stages of grief—the "Denial → Anger → Bargaining → Depression → Acceptance" cliché—but I had done it all backward. On diagnosis, I'd been prepared for death. I'd even felt good about it. I'd accepted it. I'd been ready. Then I slumped into a depression, as it became clear that I might not be dying so soon after all, which is, of course, good news, but also confusing and strangely enervating. The rapidity of the cancer science, and the nature of the statistics, meant I might live another twelve months, or another 120. Grand illnesses are supposed to be life-clarifying. Instead, I knew I was going to die—but I'd known that before. My state of knowledge was the same, but my ability to make lunch plans had been shot to hell. The way forward would seem obvious, if only I knew how many months or years I had left. Tell me three months, I'd spend time with family. Tell me one year, I'd write a book. Give me ten years, I'd get back to treating diseases. The truth that you live one day at a time didn't help: What was I supposed to do with that day?

At some point, then, I began to do a little bargaining—or not exactly bargaining. More like: "God, I have read Job, and I don't understand it, but if this is a test of faith, you now realize my faith is fairly weak, and probably leaving the spicy mustard off the pastrami sandwich would have also tested it? You didn't have to go nuclear on me, you know . . ." Then, after the bargaining, came flashes of anger: "I work my whole life to get to this point, and then you give me cancer?"

And now, finally, maybe I had arrived at denial. Maybe total denial. Maybe, in the absence of any certainty, we should just assume that we're going to live a long time. Maybe that's the only way forward.

I was operating until late at night or into the early morning, fixated on graduation, my diagnosis nine months in the past. My body was taking a beating. I was too tired to eat when I got home. I had been slowly upping the dose of Tylenol and NSAIDs and antiemetics. I had developed a persistent cough, presumably caused by scarring from the dead tumor in my lungs. I only had to keep up this relentless pace for a couple more months, I told myself, and then I would graduate from residency and settle into the comparatively calmer role of a professor.

In February, I flew to Wisconsin for a job interview. They were offering everything I wanted: millions of dollars to start a neuroscience lab, head of my own clinical service, flexibility if I needed it for my health, a tenure-track professorship, appealing job options for Lucy, high salary, beautiful scenery, idyllic town, the perfect boss. "I understand about your health, and you probably have a strong connection with your oncologist," the department chairman told me. "So if you want to keep your care there, we can fly you back and forth—though we do have a top-notch cancer center here, if you want to explore it. Is there anything else I can do to make this job more attractive?"

I thought about what Emma had told me. I had gone from being unable to believe I could be a surgeon to being one, a transformation that carried the force of religious conversion. She had always kept this part of my identity in mind, even when I couldn't. She had done what I had challenged myself to do as a doctor years earlier: accepted mortal responsibility for my soul and returned me to a point where I could return to myself. I had attained the heights of the neurosurgical trainee, set to become not only a neurosurgeon but a surgeon-scientist. Every trainee aspires to this goal; almost none make it.

That night, the chairman was driving me back to my hotel after dinner. He stopped the car and pulled over. "Let me show you something," he said. We got out and stood in front of the hospital, looking over a frozen lake, its far edge luminous with specks of light leaking from faculty houses. "In summer, you can swim or sail to work. In winter, you can ski or ice-skate."

It was like a fantasy. And in that moment, it hit me: it *was* a fantasy. We could never move to Wisconsin. What if I had a serious relapse in two years? Lucy would be isolated, stripped of her friends and family, alone, caring for a dying husband and new child. As furiously as I had tried to resist it, I realized that cancer had changed the calculus. For the last several months, I had striven with every ounce to restore my life to its precancer trajectory, trying to deny cancer any purchase on my life. As desperately as I now wanted to feel triumphant, instead I felt the claws of the crab holding me back. The curse of cancer created a strange and strained existence, challenging me to be neither blind to, nor bound by, death's approach. Even when the cancer was in retreat, it cast long shadows.

When I'd first lost the professorship at Stanford, I'd consoled myself with the idea that running a lab made sense only on a twenty-year time scale. Now I saw that this was, in fact, true. Freud started his career as a successful neuroscientist. When he realized neuroscience would need at least a century to catch up with his true ambition of understanding the mind, he set aside his microscope. I think I felt something similar. Transforming neurosurgery through my research was a gamble whose odds had been made too long by my diagnosis; the lab wasn't the place I wanted to plunk the remainder of my chips.

I could hear Emma's voice again: *You have to figure out what's most important to you.*

If I no longer sought to fly on the highest trajectory of neurosurgeon and neuroscientist, what did I want?

To be a father?

To be a neurosurgeon?

To teach?

I didn't know. But if I did not know what I wanted, I had learned something, something not found in Hippocrates, Maimonides, or Osler: the physician's duty is not to stave off death or return patients to their old lives, but to take into our arms a patient and family whose lives have disintegrated and work until they can stand back up and face, and make sense of, their own existence.

My own hubris as a surgeon stood naked to me now: as much as I focused on my responsibility and power over patients' lives, it was at best a temporary responsibility, a fleeting power. Once an acute crisis has been resolved, the patient awakened, extubated, and then discharged, the patient and family go on living—and things are never quite the same. A physician's words can ease the mind, just as the neurosurgeon's scalpel can ease a disease of the brain. Yet their uncertainties and morbidities, whether emotional or physical, remain to be grappled with.

Emma hadn't given me back my old identity. She'd protected my ability to forge a new one. And, finally, I knew I would have to.

...

On a crystalline spring morning on the third Sunday of Lent, Lucy and I went to church with my parents, who had flown in from Arizona for a weekend visit. We sat together in a long wooden pew, and my mother struck up a conversation with the family sitting next to us, first complimenting the mother on her baby daughter's eyes, then quickly moving on to matters of greater substance, her skills as a listener, confidante, and connector fully evident. During the pastor's Scripture reading, I suddenly found myself chuckling. It featured a frustrated Jesus whose metaphorical language receives literal interpretation from his followers:

Jesus answered and said to her, "Everyone who drinks this water will be thirsty again; but whoever drinks the water I shall give will never thirst; the water I shall give will become in him a spring of water welling up to eternal life." The woman said to him, "Sir, give me this water, so that I may not be thirsty or have to keep coming here to draw water."

. . . Meanwhile, the disciples urged him, "Rabbi, eat." But he said to them, "I have food to eat of which you do not know." So the disciples said to one another, "Could someone have brought him something to eat?"

It was passages like these, where there is a clear mocking of literalist readings of Scripture, that had brought me back around to Christianity after a long stretch, following college, when my notion of God and Jesus had grown, to put it gently, tenuous. During my sojourn in ironclad atheism, the primary arsenal leveled against Christianity had been its failure on empirical grounds. Surely enlightened reason offered a more coherent cosmos. Surely Occam's razor cut the faithful free from blind faith. There is no proof of God; therefore, it is unreasonable to *believe* in God.

Although I had been raised in a devout Christian family, where prayer and Scripture readings were a nightly ritual, I, like most scientific types, came to believe in the possibility of a material conception of reality, an ultimately scientific worldview that would grant a complete metaphysics, minus outmoded concepts like souls, God, and bearded white men in robes. I spent a good chunk of my twenties trying to build a frame for such an endeavor. The problem, however, eventually became evident: to make science the arbiter of metaphysics is to banish not only God from the world but also love, hate, meaning—to consider a world that is self-evidently *not* the world we live in. That's not to say that if you believe in meaning, you must also believe in God. It is to say, though, that if you believe that science provides no basis for God, then you are almost obligated to conclude that science provides no basis for meaning and, therefore, life itself doesn't have any. In other words, existential claims have no weight; all knowledge is scientific knowledge.

Yet the paradox is that scientific methodology is the product of human hands and thus cannot reach some permanent truth. We build scientific theories to organize and manipulate the world, to reduce phenomena into manageable units. Science is based on reproducibility and manufactured objectivity. As strong as that makes its ability to generate claims about matter and energy, it also makes scientific knowledge inapplicable to the existential, visceral nature of human life, which is unique and subjective and unpredictable. Science may provide the most useful way to organize empirical, reproducible data, but its power to do so is predicated on its inability to grasp the most central aspects of human life: hope, fear, love, hate, beauty, envy, honor, weakness, striving, suffering, virtue.

Between these core passions and scientific theory, there will always be a gap. No system of thought can contain the fullness of human experience. The realm of metaphysics remains the province of revelation (this, not atheism, is what Occam argued, after all). And atheism can be justified only on these grounds. The prototypical atheist, then, is Graham Greene's commandant from *The Power and the Glory*, whose atheism comes from a revelation of the absence of God. The only real atheism must be grounded in a world-making vision. The favorite quote of many an atheist, from the Nobel Prize–winning French biologist Jacques Monod, belies this revelatory aspect: "The ancient covenant is in pieces; man at last knows that he is alone in the unfeeling immensity of the universe, out of which he emerged only by chance."

Yet I returned to the central values of Christianity—sacrifice, redemption, forgiveness—because I found them so compelling. There is a tension in the Bible between justice and mercy, between the Old Testament and the New Testament. And the New Testament says you can never be good enough: goodness is the thing, and you can never live up to it. The main message of Jesus, I believed, is that mercy trumps justice every time.

Not only that, but maybe the basic message of original sin isn't "Feel guilty all the time." Maybe it is more along these lines: "We all have a notion of what it means to be good, and we can't live up to it all the time." Maybe that's what the message of the New Testament is, after all. Even if you have a notion as well defined as Leviticus, you can't live that way. It's not just impossible, it's insane.

About God I could say nothing definitive, of course, but the basic reality of human life stands compellingly against blind determinism. Moreover, no one, myself included, credits revelation with any epistemic authority. We are all reasonable people—revelation is not good enough. Even if God spoke to us, we'd discount it as delusional.

So what, I wonder, is the aspiring metaphysician to do?

Give up?

Almost.

Struggle toward the capital-T Truth, but recognize that the task is impossible—or that if a correct answer is possible, verification certainly is impossible.

In the end, it cannot be doubted that each of us can see only a part of the picture. The doctor sees one, the patient another, the engineer a third, the economist a fourth, the pearl diver a fifth, the alcoholic a sixth, the cable guy a seventh, the sheep farmer an eighth, the Indian beggar a ninth, the pastor a tenth. Human knowledge is never contained in one person. It grows from the relationships we create between each other and the world, and still it is never complete. And Truth comes somewhere above all of them, where, as at the end of that Sunday's reading, the sower and reaper can rejoice together. For here the saying is verified that "One sows and another reaps." I sent you to reap what you have not worked for; others have done the work, and you are sharing the fruits of their work.

I hopped out of the CT scanner, seven months since I had returned to surgery. This would be my last scan before finishing residency, before becoming a father, before my future became real.

"Wanna take a look, Doc?" the tech said.

"Not right now," I said. "I've got a lot of work to do today."

It was already six P.M. I had to go see patients, organize tomorrow's OR schedule, review films, dictate my clinic notes, check on my post-ops, and so on. Around eight P.M., I sat down in the neurosurgery office, next to a radiology viewing station. I turned it on, looked at my patients' scans for the next day—two simple spine cases—and, finally, typed in my own name. I zipped through the images as if they were a kid's flip-book, comparing the new scan to the last. Everything looked the same, the old tumors remained exactly the same . . . except, wait.

I rolled back the images. Looked again.

There it was. A new tumor, large, filling my right middle lobe. It looked, oddly, like a full moon having almost cleared the horizon. Going back to the old images, I could make out the faintest trace of it, a ghostly harbinger now brought fully into the world.

I was neither angry nor scared. It simply was. It was a fact about the world, like the distance from the sun to the earth. I drove home and told Lucy. It was a Thursday night, and we wouldn't see Emma again until Monday, but Lucy and I sat down in the living room, with our laptops, and mapped out the next steps: biopsies, tests, chemotherapy. The treatments this time around would be tougher to endure, the possibility of a long life more remote. Eliot again: "But at my back in a cold blast I hear / the rattle of the bones, and chuckle spread from ear to ear." Neurosurgery would be impossible for a couple of weeks, perhaps months, perhaps forever. But we decided that all of that could wait to be real until Monday. Today was Thursday, and I'd already made tomorrow's OR assignments; I planned on having one last day as a resident.

As I stepped out of my car at the hospital at five-twenty the next morning, I inhaled deeply, smelling the eucalyptus and ... was that pine? Hadn't noticed that before. I met the resident team, assembled for morning rounds. We reviewed overnight events, new admissions, new scans, then went to see our patients before M&M, or morbidity and mortality conference, a regular meeting in which the neurosurgeons gathered to review mistakes that had been made and cases that had gone wrong. Afterward, I spent an extra couple of minutes with a patient, Mr. R. He had developed a rare syndrome, called Gerstmann's, where, after I'd removed his brain tumor, he'd begun showing several specific deficits: an inability to write, to name fingers, to do arithmetic, to tell left from right. I'd seen it only once before, as a medical student eight years ago, on one of the first patients I'd followed on the neurosurgical service. Like him, Mr. R was euphoric—I wondered if that was part of the syndrome that no one had described before. Mr. R was getting better, though: his speech had returned almost to normal, and his arithmetic was only slightly off. He'd likely make a full recovery.

The morning passed, and I scrubbed for my last case. Suddenly the moment felt enormous. My last time scrubbing? Perhaps this was it. I watched the suds drip off my arms, then down the drain. I entered the OR, gowned up, and draped the patient, making sure the corners were sharp and neat. I wanted this case to be perfect. I opened the skin of his lower back. He was an elderly man whose spine had degenerated, compressing his nerve roots and causing severe pain. I pulled away the fat until the fascia appeared and I could feel the tips of his vertebrae. I opened the fascia and smoothly dissected the muscle away, until only the wide, glistening vertebrae showed up through the wound, clean and bloodless. The attending wandered in as I began to remove the lamina, the back wall of the vertebrae, whose bony overgrowths, along with ligaments beneath, were compressing the nerves.

"Looks good," he said. "If you want to go to today's conference, I can have the fellow come in and finish."

My back was beginning to ache. Why hadn't I taken an extra dose of NSAIDs beforehand? This case should be quick, though. I was almost there.

"Naw," I said. "I want to finish the case."

The attending scrubbed in, and together we completed the bony removal. He began to pick away at the ligaments, beneath which lay the dura, which contained spinal fluid and the nerve roots. The most common error at this stage is tearing a hole in the dura. I worked on the opposite side. Out of the corner of my eye, I saw near his instrument a flash of blue—the dura starting to peek through.

"Watch out!" I said, just as the mouth of his instrument bit into the dura. Clear spinal fluid began to fill the wound. I hadn't had a leak in one of my cases in more than a year. Repairing it would take another hour.

"Get the micro set out," I said. "We have a leak."

By the time we finished the repair and removed the compressive soft tissue, my shoulders burned. The attending broke scrub, offered his apologies and said his thanks, and left me to close. The layers came together nicely. I began to suture the skin, using a running nylon stitch. Most surgeons used staples, but I was convinced that nylon had lower infection rates, and we would do this one, this final closure, my way. The skin came together perfectly, without tension, as if there had been no surgery at all.

Good. One good thing.

As we uncovered the patient, the scrub nurse, one with whom I hadn't worked before, said, "You on call this weekend, Doc?"

"Nope." *And possibly never again.*

"Got any more cases today?"

"Nope." *And possibly never again.*

"Shit, well, I guess that means this is a happy ending! Work's done. I like happy endings, don't you, Doc?"

"Yeah. Yeah, I like happy endings."

I sat down by the computer to enter orders as the nurses cleaned and the anesthesiologists began to wake the patient. I had always jokingly threatened that when I was in charge, instead of the high-energy pop music everyone liked to play in the OR, we'd listen exclusively to bossa nova. I put *Getz/Gilberto* on the radio, and the soft, sonorous sounds of a saxophone filled the room.

I left the OR shortly after, then gathered my things, which had accumulated over seven years of work—extra sets of clothes for the nights you don't leave, toothbrushes, bars of soap, phone chargers, snacks, my skull model and collection of neurosurgery books, and so on.

On second thought, I left my books behind. They'd be of more use here.

On my way out to the parking lot, a fellow approached to ask me something, but his pager went off. He looked at it, waved, turned, and ran back in to the hospital—"I'll catch you later!" he called over his shoulder. Tears welled up as I sat in the car, turned the key, and slowly pulled out into the street. I drove home, walked through the front door, hung up my white coat, and took off my ID badge. I pulled the battery out of my pager. I peeled off my scrubs and took a long shower.

Later that night, I called Victoria and told her I wouldn't be in on Monday, or possibly ever again, and wouldn't be setting the OR schedule.

"You know, I've been having this recurring nightmare that this day was coming," she said. "I don't know how you did this for so long."

Lucy and I met with Emma on Monday. She confirmed the plan we'd envisioned: bronchoscopic biopsy, look for targetable mutations, otherwise chemo. The real reason

I was there, though, was for her guidance. I told her I was taking leave from neurosurgery.

"Okay," she said. "That's fine. You can stop neurosurgery if, say, you want to focus on something that matters more to you. But *not* because you are sick. You aren't any sicker than you were a week ago. This is a bump in the road, but you can keep your current trajectory. Neurosurgery was important to you."

Once again, I had traversed the line from doctor to patient, from actor to acted upon, from subject to direct object. My life up until my illness could be understood as the linear sum of my choices. As in most modern narratives, a character's fate depended on human actions, his and others. *King Lear*'s Gloucester may complain about human fate as "flies to wanton boys," but it's Lear's vanity that sets in motion the dramatic arc of the play. From the Enlightenment onward, the individual occupied center stage. But now I lived in a different world, a more ancient one, where human action paled against superhuman forces, a world that was more Greek tragedy than Shakespeare. No amount of effort can help Oedipus and his parents escape their fates; their only access to the forces controlling their lives is through the oracles and seers, those given divine vision. What I had come for was not a treatment plan—I had read enough to know the medical ways forward—but the comfort of oracular wisdom.

"This is not the end," she said, a line she must have used a thousand times—after all, did I not use similar speeches to my own patients?—to those seeking impossible answers. "Or even the beginning of the end. This is just the end of the beginning."

And I felt better.

A week after the biopsy, Alexis, the nurse practitioner, called. There were no new targetable mutations, so chemotherapy was the only option, and it was being set up for Monday. I asked about the specific agents and was told I'd have to talk to Emma. She was en route to Lake Tahoe with her kids, but she'd give me a call over the weekend.

The next day, a Saturday, Emma called. I asked her what she thought about chemotherapy agents.

"Well," she said. "Do you have specific thoughts?"

"I guess the main question is whether to include Avastin," I said. "I know the data is mixed and that it adds potential side effects, and some cancer centers are turning away from it. In my mind, though, since there are a lot of studies supporting its use, I'd lean toward including it. We can discontinue it if I have a bad reaction to it. If that seems sensible to you."

"Yeah, that sounds about right. Insurance companies also make it hard to add it later, so that's another reason to use it up front."

"Thanks for calling. I'll let you get back to enjoying the lake."

"Okay. But there's one thing." She paused. "I'm totally happy for us to make your medical plan together; obviously, you're a doctor, you know what you're talking about, and it's your life. But if you ever want me to just *be* the doctor, I'm happy to do that, too."

I hadn't ever considered that I could release myself from the responsibility of my own medical care. I'd just assumed all patients became experts at their own diseases. I remembered how, as a green medical student, knowing nothing, I would often end up asking patients to explain their diseases and treatments to me, their blue toes and pink pills. But as a doctor, I never expected patients to make decisions alone; I bore responsibility for the patient. And I realized I was trying to do the same thing now, my doctor-self remaining responsible for my patient-self. Maybe I'd been cursed by a Greek god, but abdicating control seemed irresponsible, if not impossible.

Chemotherapy began on Monday. Lucy, my mother, and I went to the infusion center together. I had an IV placed, settled into an easy chair, and waited. The drug cocktail would take four and a half hours to infuse. I passed the time napping, reading, and sometimes blankly staring, with Lucy and my mother next to me, interrupting the silence with occasional small talk. The other occupants of the room were in various states of health—some bald, some well-coiffed, some withered, some sprightly, some disheveled, some dapper. All lay still, silent, with IV tubing dripping poison into outstretched arms. I was to return every three weeks for treatment.

I began to feel the effects the next day, a deep fatigue, a profound bone-weariness setting in. Eating, normally a source of great pleasure, was like drinking seawater. Suddenly, all of my joys were salted. For breakfast, Lucy made me a bagel with cream cheese; it tasted like a salt lick. I set it aside. Reading was exhausting. I had agreed to write a few chapters on the therapeutic potential of my research with V for two major neurosurgical textbooks. That, too, I set aside. The days passed, television and forced feedings marking the time. A pattern developed over the weeks: the malaise would slowly ease, normalcy returning just in time for the next treatment.

The cycles continued; I shuffled in and out of the hospital with minor complications, which were just enough to preclude any return to work. The neurosurgery department determined that I had met all national and local criteria for graduation; the ceremony was scheduled for a Saturday, about two weeks before Lucy's due date.

The day arrived. As I stood in our bedroom, dressing for graduation—the culmination of seven years of residency—a piercing nausea struck me. This was unlike the usual nausea of chemotherapy, which washed over you like a wave and, like a wave, could be ridden. I began uncontrollably vomiting green bile, its chalky taste distinct from stomach acid. This was from deep in my gut.

I would not be going to graduation, after all.

I needed IV fluids to avoid dehydration, so Lucy

drove me to the emergency department and rehydration began. The vomiting gave way to diarrhea. The medical resident, Brad, and I chatted amicably, and I relayed my medical history, covering all my medications, and we ended up discussing advances in molecular therapies, especially Tarceva, which I was still taking. The medical plan was simple: keep me hydrated with intravenous fluids until I could drink enough by mouth. That evening, I was admitted to a hospital room. But when the nurse reviewed my medication list, I noticed Tarceva was not on it. I asked her to call the resident to correct the oversight. These things happen. I was taking a dozen medications, after all. Keeping track was not easy.

It was well past midnight when Brad appeared.

"I heard you had a question about your medications?" he asked.

"Yeah," I said. "Tarceva wasn't ordered. Do you mind ordering it?"

"I decided to take you off it."

"Why is that?"

"Your liver enzymes are too high to take it."

I was confused. My liver enzymes had been high for months; if this was an issue, why hadn't we discussed it before? In any case, this was clearly a mistake. "Emma—my oncologist, your boss—has seen these numbers, and she wants to keep me on it."

Residents routinely have to make medical decisions without the attending's input. But now that he had Emma's opinion, surely he would capitulate.

"But it might be causing your GI problems."

My confusion deepened. Usually invoking the attending's orders ends the discussion. "I've been taking it for a year without any problems," I said. "You think Tarceva is causing this all of a sudden, and not the chemotherapy?"

"Maybe, yeah."

Confusion yielded to anger. Some kid two years out of med school, no older than my junior residents, was really arguing with me? It'd be one thing if he were right, but he wasn't making any sense. "Um, didn't I mention this afternoon that without that pill, my bone metastases become active and produce excruciating pain? I don't mean to sound dramatic, but I've broken bones boxing, and this is far more painful. As in, ten-out-of-ten pain. As in, I-Will-Actually-Soon-Be-Screaming pain."

"Well, given the half-life of the drug, that probably won't happen for a day or so."

I could see that in Brad's eyes I was not a patient, I was a problem: a box to be checked off.

"Look," he continued, "if you weren't you, we wouldn't even be having this conversation. I'd just stop the drug and make you prove it causes all this pain."

What had happened to our amicable chat this afternoon? I thought back to med school, when a patient had told me that she always wore her most expensive socks to the doctor's office, so that when she was in a patient's gown and shoeless, the doctor would see the socks and know she was a person of substance, to be treated with respect. (Ah, there's the problem—I was wearing hospital-issue socks, which I had been stealing for years!)

"Anyway, Tarceva is a special drug, and it requires a fellow or attending to sign off on it. Do you really want me to wake someone up for this? Can't it wait till morning?"

And there it was.

Meeting his obligation to me meant adding one more thing to his to-do list: an embarrassing phone call with his boss, revealing his error. He was working the night shift. Residency education regulations had forced most programs to adopt shift work. And along with shift work comes a kind of shiftiness, a subtle undercutting of responsibility. If he could just push it off for a few more hours, I would become somebody else's problem.

"I usually take it at five A.M.," I said. "And you know as well as I do that 'waiting till morning' means letting someone deal with it after morning rounds, which will be more like the afternoon. Right?"

"Okay, fine," he said, and left the room.

When morning arrived, I discovered that he had not ordered the medication.

Emma dropped in to say hello and told me she would sort out the Tarceva order. She wished me a speedy recovery and apologized for the fact that she was heading out of town for a week. Over the course of the day I began to deteriorate, my diarrhea rapidly worsening. I was being rehydrated, but not quickly enough. My kidneys began to fail. My mouth became so dry I could not speak or swallow. At the next lab check, my serum sodium had reached a near-fatal level. I was transferred to the ICU. Part of my soft palate and pharynx died from dehydration and peeled out of my mouth. I was in pain, floating through varying levels of consciousness, while a pantheon of specialists was brought together to help: medical intensivists, nephrologists, gastroenterologists, endocrinologists, infectious disease specialists, neuro-surgeons, general oncologists, thoracic oncologists, otolaryngologists. Lucy, thirty-eight weeks pregnant, stayed with me by day and secretly moved into my old call room, steps from the ICU, so she could check on me at night. She and my father also lent their voices.

During lucid moments, I was acutely aware that with this many voices, cacophony results. In medicine, this is known as the WICOS problem: Who Is the Captain Of the Ship? The nephrologists disagreed with the ICU doctors, who disagreed with the endocrinologists, who disagreed with the oncologists, who disagreed with the gastroenterologists. I felt the responsibility of my care: during bouts of consciousness, I typed out the sequential details of my current illness and, with Lucy's help, tried to corral all the doctors to keep the facts and interpreta-tions straight. Later, while half asleep, I could dimly hear my father and Lucy discussing my condition with each team of doctors. We suspected that the main plan should

"I'm not sure that's something you can find by read-ing about it," she replied.

Emma was now the captain of the ship, lending a sense of calm to the chaos of this hospitalization. T. S. Eliot sprang to mind:

> *Damyata:* The boat responded
> Gaily, to the hand expert with sail and oar
> The sea was calm, your heart would have
>   responded
> Gaily, when invited, beating obedient
> To controlling hands

I leaned back in my hospital bed and closed my eyes. As the darkness of delirium descended again, I finally re-laxed.

Lucy's due date came and went without labor, and I was finally scheduled to be discharged from the hospital. I had lost over forty pounds since being diagnosed, fifteen in the last week. I weighed as much as I had in eighth grade, though my hair had considerably thinned since those days, mostly in the past month. I was awake again, alert to the world, but withered. I could see my bones against my skin, a living X-ray. At home, simply holding my head up was tiring. Lifting a glass of water required both hands. Reading was out of the question.

Both sets of parents were in town to help. Two days after discharge, Lucy had her first contractions. She stayed home while my mother drove me to my follow-up appointment with Emma.

"Frustrated?" Emma asked.

"No."

"You should be. It's going to be a long recovery."

"Well, yes, okay. I am frustrated on the big picture. But on the day-by-day, I'm ready to get back to physical therapy and start recovering. I did it once, so it should be old hat, right?"

"Did you see your last scan?" she asked.

"No, I've kind of stopped looking."

"It looks good," she said. "The disease looks stable, maybe even slightly shrinking."

We talked through some of the coming logistics; chemotherapy would be on hold until I was stronger. Experimental trials wouldn't accept me in my current state, either. Treatment wasn't an option—not until I regained some strength. I leaned my head against the wall to support the flagging muscles of my neck. My thoughts were clouded. I needed that oracle to scry again, to gather secrets from birds or star charts, from mutant genes or Kaplan-Meier graphs.

"Emma," I said, "what's the next step?"

"Get stronger. That's it."

"But when the cancer recurs ... I mean, the probabilities ..." I paused. First-line therapy (Tarceva) had failed. Second-line therapy (chemo) had nearly killed me. Third-line therapy, if I could even get there, made few promises. Beyond that, the vast unknown of experimental treatments. Phrases of doubt fell from my mouth. "I mean, getting back to the OR, or to walking, or even—"

"You have five good years left," she said.

She pronounced it, but without the authoritative tone of an oracle, without the confidence of a true believer. She said it, instead, like a plea. Like that patient who could speak only in numbers. Like she was not so much speaking to me as pleading, a mere human, with whatever forces and fates truly control these things. There we were, doctor and patient, in a relationship that some-times carries a magisterial air and other times, like now, was no more, and no less, than two people huddled to-gether, as one faces the abyss.

Doctors, it turns out, need hope, too.

On the way home from the appointment with Emma, Lucy's mom called to say they were headed to the hospital. Lucy was in labor. ("Make sure you ask about the epidural early," I told her. She had suffered enough.) I returned to the hospital, pushed by my father in a wheelchair. I lay down on a cot in the delivery room, heat packs and blankets keeping my skeletal body from shivering. For the next two hours, I watched Lucy and the nurse go through the ritual of labor. As a contraction built up, the nurse counted off the pushing: "And a one two three four five six seven eight nine and a ten!"

Lucy turned to me, smiling. "It feels like I'm playing a sport!" she said.

I lay on the cot and smiled back, watching her belly rise. There would be so many absences in Lucy's and my daughter's life—if this was as present as I could be, then so be it.

Sometime after midnight, the nurse nudged me awake. "It's almost time," she whispered. She gathered the blankets and helped me to a chair, next to Lucy. The obstetrician was already in the room, no older than I. She looked up at me as the baby was crowning. "I can tell you one thing: your daughter has hair exactly like yours," she said. "And a lot of it." I nodded, holding Lucy's hand during the last moments of her labor. And then, with one final push, on July 4, at 2:11 A.M., there she was. Elizabeth Acadia—Cady; we had picked the name months before.

"Can we put her on your skin, Papa?" the nurse asked me.

"No, I'm too c-c-cold," I said, my teeth chattering. "But I would love to hold her."

They wrapped her in blankets and handed her to me. Feeling her weight in one arm, and gripping Lucy's hand with the other, the possibilities of life emanated before us. The cancer cells in my body would still be dying, or they'd start growing again. Looking out over the expanse ahead I saw not an empty wasteland but something simpler: a blank page on which I would go on.

Yet there is dynamism in our house.

Day to day, week to week, Cady blossoms: a first grasp, a first smile, a first laugh. Her pediatrician regularly records her growth on charts, tick marks indicating her progress over time. A brightening newness surrounds her. As she sits in my lap smiling, enthralled by my tuneless singing, an incandescence lights the room.

Time for me is now double-edged: every day brings me further from the low of my last relapse but closer to the next recurrence—and, eventually, death. Perhaps later than I think, but certainly sooner than I desire. There are, I imagine, two responses to that realization. The most obvious might be an impulse to frantic activity: to "live life to its fullest," to travel, to dine, to achieve a host of neglected ambitions. Part of the cruelty of cancer, though, is not only that it limits your time; it also limits your energy, vastly reducing the amount you can squeeze into a day. It is a tired hare who now races. And even if I had the energy, I prefer a more tortoiselike approach. I plod, I ponder. Some days, I simply persist.

If time dilates when one moves at high speeds, does it contract when one moves barely at all? It must: the days have shortened considerably.

With little to distinguish one day from the next, time has begun to feel static. In English, we use the word *time* in different ways: "The time is two forty-five" versus "I'm going through a tough time." These days, time feels less like the ticking clock and more like a state of being. Languor settles in. There's a feeling of openness. As a surgeon, focused on a patient in the OR, I might have found the position of the clock's hands arbitrary, but I never thought them meaningless. Now the time of day means nothing, the day of the week scarcely more. Medical training is relentlessly future-oriented, all about delayed gratification; you're always thinking about what you'll be doing five years down the line. But now I don't know what I'll be doing five years down the line. I may be dead. I may not be. I may be healthy. I may be writing. I don't know. And so it's not all that useful to spend time thinking about the future—that is, beyond lunch.

Verb conjugation has become muddled, as well.

Which is correct: "I am a neurosurgeon," "I was a neuro-surgeon," or "I had been a neurosurgeon before and will be again"? Graham Greene once said that life was lived in the first twenty years and the remainder was just re-flection. So what tense am I living in now? Have I pro-ceeded beyond the present tense and into the past perfect? The future tense seems vacant and, on others' lips, jarring. A few months ago, I celebrated my fifteenth college reunion at Stanford and stood out on the quad, drinking a whiskey as a pink sun dipped below the hori-zon; when old friends called out parting promises—"We'll see you at the twenty-fifth!"—it seemed rude to respond with "Well . . . probably not."

Everyone succumbs to finitude. I suspect I am not the only one who reaches this pluperfect state. Most am-bitions are either achieved or abandoned; either way, they belong to the past. The future, instead of the ladder toward the goals of life, flattens out into a perpetual present. Money, status, all the vanities the preacher of Ecclesiastes described hold so little interest: a chasing after wind, indeed.

Yet one thing cannot be robbed of her futurity: our daughter, Cady. I hope I'll live long enough that she has some memory of me. Words have a longevity I do not. I had thought I could leave her a series of letters—but what would they say? I don't know what this girl will be like when she is fifteen; I don't even know if she'll take to the nickname we've given her. There is perhaps only one thing to say to this infant, who is all future, overlapping briefly with me, whose life, barring the improbable, is all but past.

That message is simple:

When you come to one of the many moments in life where you must give an account of yourself, provide a ledger of what you have been, and done, and meant to the world, do not, I pray, discount that you filled a dying man's days with a sated joy, a joy unknown to me in all my prior years, a joy that does not hunger for more and more but rests, satisfied. In this time, right now, that is an enormous thing.

EPILOGUE

Lucy Kalanithi

You left me, sweet, two legacies,—
A legacy of love
A Heavenly Father would content,
Had he the offer of;

You left me boundaries of pain
Capacious as the sea,
Between eternity and time,
Your consciousness and me.

—Emily Dickinson

PAUL DIED ON MONDAY, March 9, 2015, surrounded by his family, in a hospital bed roughly two hundred yards from the labor and delivery ward where our daughter, Cady, had entered the world eight months before. Between Cady's birth and Paul's death, if you'd seen us sucking on ribs at our local barbecue restaurant and smiling over a shared beer, a dark-haired baby with long eyelashes napping in her stroller beside us, you'd never have guessed that Paul likely had less than a year to live, nor that we understood that.

It was around Cady's first Christmas, when she was five months old, that Paul's cancer began to resist the third-line drugs recommended after Tarceva and then chemotherapy had stopped working. Cady tried her first solid food during that holiday season, snug in candy-cane-striped pajamas, gumming mashed yams as family gathered at Paul's childhood home in Kingman, Arizona, the house aglow with candles and chatter. His strength waned over the following months, but we continued to experience joyful moments, even in the midst of our sorrow. We hosted cozy dinner parties, held each other at night, and delighted in our daughter's bright eyes and calm nature. And, of course, Paul wrote, reclining in his armchair, wrapped in a warm fleece blanket. In his final months, he was singularly focused on finishing this book.

As winter turned to spring, the saucer magnolias in our neighborhood bloomed large and pink, but Paul's health was declining rapidly. By late February, he needed supplemental oxygen to keep his breathing comfortable. I was adding his untouched lunch to the trash can atop his untouched breakfast, and a few hours later I'd add an untouched dinner to the pile. He used to love my breakfast sandwiches—egg, sausage, and cheese on a roll—but with his waning appetite we'd changed to eggs and toast, then just eggs, until even those became intolerable. Even his favorite smoothies, the glasses I filled with a steady stream of calories, were unappetizing.

Bedtime crept earlier, Paul's voice slurred intermittently, and his nausea became unremitting. A CT scan and brain MRI confirmed worsening cancer in Paul's lungs and new tumors that had landed in his brain, including leptomeningeal carcinomatosis, a rare and lethal infiltration that brought with it a prognosis of only several months and the looming shadow of swift neurologic decline. The news hit Paul hard. He said little, but as a neurosurgeon, he knew what lay ahead. Although Paul accepted his limited life expectancy, neurologic decline was a new devastation, the prospect of losing meaning and agency agonizing. We strategized with Paul's oncologist about his top priority: preserving mental acuity as long as possible. We arranged entry into a clinical trial, consultation with a neuro-oncology specialist, and a visit with his palliative-care team to discuss hospice the medication. Therefore, Paul's oncologist had instructed me to videotape him daily, doing the same task, to track any deficits in his speech or gait. "April is the cruellest month," Paul read aloud in the living room that Saturday as I filmed, choosing T. S. Eliot's *The Waste Land* as his script. "Mixing memory and desire, stirring / Dull roots with spring rain." The family chuckled when, though it was not part of the assignment, he set the book facedown on his lap and insisted on reciting from memory.

"So like him!" his mother said, smiling.

The next day, Sunday, we hoped for a continuation of the calm weekend. If Paul felt well enough, we would attend church, then take Cady and her cousin to the baby swings at the park up the hill. We'd continue to absorb the recent painful news, share the sorrow, savor our time together.

But instead, time sped up.

Early Sunday morning, I stroked Paul's forehead and found it scorching with fever, 104 degrees, though he was relatively comfortable and free of other new symptoms. We made it in and out of the emergency room within a few hours, Paul's father and Suman with us, returning home to the rest of the family after starting antibiotics in case of pneumonia (Paul's chest X-ray was dense with tumors, which could obscure an infection). But was this, instead, the cancer progressing rapidly? Paul napped comfortably in the afternoon, but he was gravely ill. I started to cry as I watched him sleep, then crept out to our living room, where his father's tears joined mine. I already missed him.

Sunday evening, Paul's condition worsened abruptly. He sat on the edge of our bed, struggling to breathe— a startling change. I called an ambulance. When we re-entered the emergency room, Paul on a gurney this time, his parents close behind us, he turned toward me and whispered, "This might be how it ends."

"I'm here with you," I said.

The hospital staff greeted Paul warmly, as always. But they moved quickly once they saw his condition. After initial testing, they placed a mask over his nose and mouth to help his breathing via BiPAP, a breathing support system that supplied a strong mechanized flow of air each time he inhaled, doing much of the work of breathing for him. Though it helps with respiratory mechanics, BiPAP can be hard work for a patient—noisy and forceful, blowing one's lips apart with each breath like those of a dog with its head out a car window. I stood close, leaning over the gurney, my hand in Paul's as the steady *whoosh, whoosh* of the machine began.

Paul's blood carbon dioxide level was critically high, indicating that the work of breathing was overwhelming him. Blood tests suggested that some of the excess carbon dioxide had been accumulating over days to weeks, as his lung disease and debility had advanced. Because his brain had slowly become acclimated to higher-than-normal levels of carbon dioxide, he remained lucid. He observed. He understood, as a physician, the ominous test results. I understood them, too, walking behind him as he was wheeled to an intensive-care room, one where so many of his own patients had struggled before or after neurosurgery, their families assembled in vinyl chairs by their bedsides. "Will I need to be intubated?" he asked me between BiPAP breaths when we arrived. "*Should* I be intubated?"

Through the night, Paul discussed that question in a series of conversations with his physicians, his family, and then just me. Around midnight, the critical-care attending, a longtime mentor to Paul, came in to discuss treatment options with the family. BiPAP was a temporary solution, he said. The only remaining intervention would be for Paul to be intubated—put on a ventilator. Was that what he wanted?

The key question quickly came into view: Could the sudden respiratory failure be reversed?

Of concern was whether Paul would remain too ill to ever come off the ventilator—would he be lost to delirium and then organ failure, first mind and then body slipping away? We'd witnessed this agonizing scenario as physicians. Paul explored the alternative: in lieu of intubation, he could choose "comfort care," though death would come more surely and swiftly. "Even if I make it through this," he said, thinking of the cancer in his brain, "I'm not sure I see a future that includes meaningful time." His mother chimed in, desperately. "No decisions tonight, Pubby," she said. "Let's all get some rest." After ensuring his "do not resuscitate" status, Paul agreed. Sympathetic nurses brought him extra blankets. I switched off the fluorescent lights.

Paul managed to doze until sunrise, his father sitting vigil while I napped briefly in an adjacent room, hoping to preserve my mental strength, knowing that the following day might be the hardest of my life. I crept back to Paul's room at six A.M., the lights still low, the intensive-care monitors chiming intermittently. Paul opened his eyes. We talked again about "comfort care"—avoiding aggressive attempts to forestall his decline—and he wondered aloud whether he could go home. He was so ill that I worried he might suffer and die on the way. However, I said I would do everything possible to take him home if that was most important to him, nodding that yes, comfort care might be the direction we were headed. Or was there some way to re-create home here? Between BiPAP puffs, he answered: "Cady."

Cady arrived in short order—our friend Victoria had retrieved her from home—and began her own unwitting, cheerful vigil, happily nestled in the crook of Paul's right arm, tugging at her tiny socks, batting at his hospital blankets, smiling and cooing, unbothered by the BiPAP machine as it continued to blow, keeping Paul alive.

The medical team came by on rounds, discussing Paul's case outside the room, where his family and I joined them. Paul's acute respiratory failure was likely rapid cancer progression. His carbon dioxide level was rising still—a hardening indication for intubation. The family was torn: Paul's oncologist had phoned in, hopeful that the acute problem could be ameliorated, but the physicians present were less optimistic. I entreated them to weigh in with as much conviction as possible on the chance of reversing his abrupt decline.

"He doesn't want a Hail Mary," I said. "If he doesn't have a chance of meaningful time, he wants to take the mask off and hold Cady."

I returned to Paul's bedside. He looked at me, his dark eyes alert above the nose bridge of the BiPAP mask, and said clearly, his voice soft but unwavering, "I'm ready."

Ready, he meant, to remove the breathing support, to start morphine, to die.

The family gathered together. During the precious minutes after Paul's decision, we all expressed our love and respect. Tears glistened in Paul's eyes. He expressed gratitude to his parents. He asked us to ensure that his manuscript be published in some form. He told me a last time that he loved me. The attending physician stepped in with strengthening words: "Paul, after you die, your family will fall apart, but they'll pull it back together because of the example of bravery you set." Jeevan's eyes were trained on Paul as Suman said, "Go in peace, my brother." With my heart breaking, I climbed into the last bed we would share.

I thought of other beds we'd shared. Eight years prior, as medical students, we'd slept similarly ensconced in a twin bed next to my grandfather as he lay dying at home, having cut our honeymoon short to help with caregiving duties. We awakened every few hours to give him medications, my love for Paul deepening as I watched him lean in and listen closely to my grandfather's whispered requests. We'd never have imagined this scene, Paul's own deathbed, so near in our future. Twenty-two months ago, we'd cried in a bed on another floor of this same hospital as we learned of Paul's cancer diagnosis. Eight months ago, we'd been together here in my hospital bed the day after Cady was born, both napping, the first good, long sleep I'd had since her birth, wrapped in each other's arms. I thought of our cozy bed empty at home, remembered falling in love in New Haven twelve years earlier, surprised right away by how well our bodies and limbs fit together, and thought of how ever since, we'd both slept best when entwined. I hoped with all I had that he felt that same restful comfort now.

An hour later, the mask and monitors were off, and morphine was flowing through Paul's IV. He was breathing steadily but shallowly, and he appeared comfortable. Nonetheless, I asked him whether he needed more morphine, and he nodded yes, his eyes closed. His mother sat close; his father's hand rested atop his head. Finally, he slipped into unconsciousness.

For more than nine hours, Paul's family—his parents, brothers, sister-in-law, daughter, and I—sat vigil as Paul, unconscious, now drew increasingly halting, infrequent breaths, his eyelids closed, his face unburdened. His long fingers rested softly in mine. Paul's parents cradled Cady and then put her in the bed again to snuggle, nurse, nap. The room, saturated with love, mirrored the many holidays and weekends we had all spent together over the years. I stroked Paul's hair, whispering, "You're a brave

Paladin"—my nickname for him—and singing quietly into his ear a favorite jingle we'd made up over the previous months, its core message being "Thank you for loving me." A close cousin and uncle arrived, and then our pastor. The family shared loving anecdotes and inside jokes; then we all took turns weeping, studying Paul's face and each other's with concern, steeped in the preciousness and pain of this time, our last hours all together.

Warm rays of evening light began to slant through the northwest-facing window of the room as Paul's breaths grew more quiet. Cady rubbed her eyes with chubby fists as her bedtime approached, and a family friend arrived to take her home. I held her cheek to Paul's, tufts of their matching dark hair similarly askew, his face serene, hers quizzical but calm, his beloved baby never suspecting that this moment was a farewell. Softly I sang Cady's bedtime song, to her, to both of them, and then released her.

As the room darkened into night, a low wall lamp glowing warmly, Paul's breaths became faltering and irregular. His body continued to appear restful, his limbs relaxed. Just before nine o'clock, his lips apart and eyes closed, Paul inhaled and then released one last, deep, final breath.

When Breath Becomes Air is, in a sense, unfinished, derailed by Paul's rapid decline, but that is an essential component of its truth, of the reality Paul faced. During the last year of his life, Paul wrote relentlessly, fueled by purpose, motivated by a ticking clock. He started with midnight bursts when he was still a neurosurgery chief resident, softly tapping away on his laptop as he lay next to me in bed; later he spent afternoons in his recliner, drafted paragraphs in his oncologist's waiting room, took phone calls from his editor while chemotherapy dripped into his veins, carried his silver laptop everywhere he went. When his fingertips developed painful fissures because of his chemotherapy, we found seamless, silver-lined gloves that allowed use of a trackpad and keyboard. Strategies for retaining the mental focus needed to write, despite the punishing fatigue of progressive cancer, were the focus of his palliative-care appointments. He was determined to keep writing.

This book carries the urgency of racing against time, of having important things to say. Paul confronted death—examined it, wrestled with it, accepted it—as a physician and a patient. He wanted to help people understand death and face their mortality. Dying in one's fourth decade is unusual now, but *dying* is not. "The thing about lung cancer is that it's not exotic," Paul wrote in an email to his best friend, Robin. "It's just tragic enough and just imaginable enough. [The reader] can get into these shoes, walk a bit, and say, 'So that's what it looks like from here . . . sooner or later I'll be back here in my own shoes.' That's what I'm aiming for, I think. Not the sensationalism of dying, and not exhortations to gather rosebuds, but: Here's what lies up ahead on the road." Of course, he did more than just describe the terrain. He traversed it bravely.

Paul's decision not to avert his eyes from death epitomizes a fortitude we don't celebrate enough in our death-avoidant culture. His strength was defined by ambition and effort, but also by softness, the opposite of bitterness. He spent much of his life wrestling with the question of how to live a meaningful life, and his book explores that essential territory. "Always the seer is a sayer," Emerson wrote. "Somehow his dream is told; somehow he publishes it with solemn joy." Writing this book was a chance for this courageous seer to be a sayer, to teach us to face death with integrity.

Most of our family and friends will have been unaware, until the publication of this book, of the marital trouble Paul and I weathered toward the end of his residency. But I am glad Paul wrote about it. It's part of our truth, another redefinition, a piece of the struggle and redemption and meaning of Paul's life and mine. His cancer diagnosis was like a nutcracker, getting us back into the soft, nourishing meat of our marriage. We hung on to each other for his physical survival and our emotional survival, our love stripped bare. We each joked to close friends that the secret to saving a relationship is for one person to become terminally ill. Conversely, we knew that one trick to managing a terminal illness is to be deeply in love—to be vulnerable, kind, generous, grateful. A few months after his diagnosis, we sang the hymn "The Servant Song" while standing side by side in a church pew, and the words vibrated with meaning as we faced uncertainty and pain together: "I will share your joy and sorrow / Till we've seen this journey through."

When Paul told me, immediately after his diagnosis, to remarry after he died, it exemplified the way he would, throughout his illness, work hard to secure my future. He was fiercely committed to ensuring the best for me, in our finances, my career, what motherhood would mean. At the same time, I worked hard to secure his present, to make his remaining time the best it could be, tracking and managing every symptom and aspect of his medical care—the most important doctoring role of my life—while supporting his ambitions, listening to his whispered fears as we embraced in the safety of our darkened bedroom, witnessing, acknowledging, accepting, comforting. We were as inseparable as we had been as medical students, when we would hold hands during lectures. Now we held hands in his coat pocket during walks outside after chemotherapy, Paul in a winter coat and hat even when the weather turned warm. He knew he would never be alone, never suffer unnecessarily. At home in bed a few weeks before he died, I asked him, "Can you breathe okay with my head on your chest like this?" His answer was "It's the only way I know how to breathe." That Paul and I formed part of the deep meaning of each other's lives is one of the greatest blessings that has ever come to me.

Both of us drew strength from Paul's family, who bolstered us as we weathered his illness and supported us in bringing our own child into the family. Despite stunning grief over their son's illness, his parents remained an unwavering source of comfort and security. Renting an apartment nearby, they visited often, Paul's father rubbing his feet, his mother making him Indian *dosa* with coconut chutney. Paul, Jeevan, and Suman lounged on our sofas, Paul's legs propped up to alleviate his back pain, discussing the "syntax" of football plays. Jeevan's wife, Emily, and I laughed nearby while Cady and her cousins, Eve and James, napped. On those afternoons, our living room felt like a small, safe village. Later in that same room, Paul would hold Cady in his writing chair, reading aloud works by Robert Frost, T. S. Eliot, Wittgenstein, as I snapped photos. Such simple moments swelled with grace and beauty, and even luck, if such a concept can be said to exist at all. And yet we did feel lucky, grateful—for family, for community, for opportunity, for our daughter, for having risen to meet each other at a time when absolute trust and acceptance were required. Although these last few years have been wrenching and difficult—sometimes almost impossible—they have also been the most beautiful and profound of my life, requiring the daily act of holding life and death, joy and pain in balance and exploring new depths of gratitude and love.

Relying on his own strength and the support of his family and community, Paul faced each stage of his illness with grace—not with bravado or a misguided faith that he would "overcome" or "beat" cancer but with an authenticity that allowed him to grieve the loss of the future he had planned and forge a new one. He cried on the day he was diagnosed. He cried while looking at a drawing we kept on the bathroom mirror that said, "I want to spend all the rest of my days here with you." He cried on his last day in the operating room. He let himself be open and vulnerable, let himself be comforted. Even while terminally ill, Paul was fully alive; despite physical collapse, he remained vigorous, open, full of hope not for an unlikely cure but for days that were full of purpose and meaning.

Paul's voice in *When Breath Becomes Air* is strong and distinctive, but also somewhat solitary. Parallel to this story are the love and warmth and spaciousness and radical permission that surrounded him. We all inhabit different selves in space and time. Here he is as a doctor, as a patient, and within a doctor-patient relationship. He wrote with a clear voice, the voice of someone with limited time, a ceaseless striver, though there were other selves as well. Not fully captured in these pages are Paul's sense of humor—he was wickedly funny—or his sweetness and tenderness, the value he placed on relationships with friends and family. But this is the book he wrote; this was his voice during this time; this was his message during this time; this was what he wrote when he needed to write it. Indeed, the version of Paul I miss most, more even than the robust, dazzling version with whom I first fell in love, is the beautiful, focused man he was in his last year, the Paul who wrote this book—frail but never weak.

Paul was proud of this book, which was a culmination of his love for literature—he once said that he found poetry more comforting than Scripture—and his ability to forge from his life a cogent, powerful tale of living with death. When Paul emailed his best friend in May 2013 to inform him that he had terminal cancer, he wrote, "The good news is I've already outlived two Brontës, Keats, and Stephen Crane. The bad news is that I haven't written anything." His journey thereafter was one of transformation—from one passionate vocation to another, from husband to father, and finally, of course, from life to death, the ultimate transformation that awaits us all. I am proud to have been his partner throughout, including while he wrote this book, an act that allowed him to live with hope, with that delicate alchemy of agency and opportunity that he writes about so eloquently, until the very end.

Paul was buried in a willow casket at the edge of a field in the Santa Cruz Mountains, overlooking the Pacific Ocean and a coastline studded with memories—brisk hikes, seafood feasts, birthday cocktails. Two months before, on a warm weekend in January, we'd dipped Cady's chubby feet into the briny water at a beach below. He was unattached to the fate of his body after he died, and he left it to us to make decisions on his behalf. I believe we chose well. Paul's grave looks west, over five miles of green hillcrests, to the ocean. Around him are hills covered in wild grass, coniferous trees, and yellow euphorbia. As you sit down, you hear wind, chirping birds, the scuffling of chipmunks. He made it here on his own terms, and his grave site feels appropriately full of ruggedness and honor, a place he deserves to be—a place we all deserve to be. I am reminded of a line from a blessing my grandfather liked: "We shall rise insensibly, and reach the tops of the everlasting hills, where the winds are cool and the sight is glorious."

And yet this is not always an easy place to be. The weather is unpredictable. Because Paul is buried on the windward side of the mountains, I have visited him in blazing sun, shrouding fog, and cold, stinging rain. It can be as uncomfortable as it is peaceful, both communal and lonely—like death, like grief—but there is beauty in all of it, and I think this is good and right.

I visit his grave often, taking a small bottle of Madeira, the wine of our honeymoon destination. Each time, I pour some out on the grass for Paul. When Paul's parents and brothers are with me, we talk as I rub the grass as if it were Paul's hair. Cady visits his grave before her nap, lying on a blanket, watching the clouds pass overhead and grabbing at the flowers we've laid down. The evening before Paul's memorial service, our siblings and I gathered with twenty of Paul's oldest, closest friends, and I wondered briefly if we'd mar the grass because we poured out so much whiskey.

Often I return to the grave after leaving flowers—tulips, lilies, carnations—to find the heads eaten by deer. It's just as good a use for the flowers as any, and one Paul would have liked. The earth is quickly turned over by worms, the processes of nature marching on, reminding me of what Paul saw and what I now carry deep in my bones, too: the inextricability of life and death, and the ability to cope, to find meaning despite this, because of this. What happened to Paul was tragic, but he was not a tragedy.

I expected to feel only empty and heartbroken after Paul died. It never occurred to me that you could love someone the same way after he was gone, that I would continue to feel such love and gratitude alongside the terrible sorrow, the grief so heavy that at times I shiver and moan under the weight of it. Paul is gone, and I miss him acutely nearly every moment, but I somehow feel

I'm still taking part in the life we created together. "Bereavement is not the truncation of married love," C. S. Lewis wrote, "but one of its regular phases—like the honeymoon. What we want is to live our marriage well and faithfully through that phase too." Caring for our daughter, nurturing relationships with family, publishing this book, pursuing meaningful work, visiting Paul's grave, grieving and honoring him, persisting . . . my love goes on—lives on—in a way I'd never expected.

When I see the hospital where Paul lived and died as a physician and a patient, I understand that had he lived, he would have made great contributions as a neurosurgeon and neuroscientist. He would have helped countless patients and their families through some of the most challenging moments of their lives, the task that drew him to neurosurgery in the first place. He was, and would have continued to be, a good person and a deep thinker. Instead, this book is a new way for him to help others, a contribution only he could make. This doesn't make his death, our loss, any less painful. But he found meaning in the striving. On page 115 of this book, he wrote, "You can't ever reach perfection, but you can believe in an asymptote toward which you are ceaselessly striving." It was arduous, bruising work, and he never faltered. This was the life he was given, and this is what he made of it. *When Breath Becomes Air* is complete, just as it is.

Two days after Paul died, I wrote a journal entry addressed to Cady: "When someone dies, people tend to say great things about him. Please know that all the wonderful things people are saying now about your dad are true. He really was that good and that brave." Reflecting on his purpose, I often think of lyrics from the hymn derived from *The Pilgrim's Progress:* "Who would true valour see, / Let him come hither . . . / Then fancies fly away, / He'll fear not what men say, / He'll labour night and day / To be a pilgrim." Paul's decision to look death in the eye was a testament not just to who he was in the final hours of his life but who he had always been. For much of his life, Paul wondered about death—and whether he could face it with integrity. In the end, the answer was yes.

I was his wife and a witness.

ACKNOWLEDGMENTS

Thank you to Dorian Karchmar, Paul's agent at William Morris Endeavor, whose fierce support and nurturing gave Paul the confidence that he could write an important book. And to Andy Ward, Paul's editor at Random House, whose determination, wisdom, and editorial talent made Paul eager to work with him, and whose humor and compassion made Paul want to befriend him. When Paul asked his family—literally his dying wish—to shepherd this book to publication posthumously, I was able to promise him that we would, because of our shared confidence in Dorian and Andy. At that time, the manuscript was just an open file on his computer, but thanks to their talent and dedication, I believe Paul died knowing that these words would make their way into the world and that, through them, our daughter would come to know him. Thank you to Abraham Verghese for a foreword that would have thrilled Paul (my only objection being that what Dr. Verghese judged to be a "prophet's beard" was really an "I-don't-have-time-to-shave" beard!). I am grateful to Emily Rapp for her willingness to meet me in my grief and coach me through the epilogue, teaching me, as Paul did, what a writer is and why writers write. Thank you to all who have supported our family, including the readers of this book. Finally, thank you to the advocates, clinicians, and scientists working tirelessly to advance lung cancer awareness and research, aiming to turn even advanced lung cancer into a survivable disease.

Lucy Kalanithi